Capnography in Clinical Practice

Pat ESCANDON, MD

J.S. Gravenstein, M.D., Dr. h.c.
Graduate Research Professor of Anesthesiology
College of Medicine
University of Florida
Gainesville, FL

David A. Paulus, M.D., M.S.
Associate Professor of Anesthesiology and Mechanical
  Engineering
Colleges of Medicine and Engineering
University of Florida
Gainesville, FL

Thomas J. Hayes, B.S.
Product Manager
Waltham Division
Hewlett Packard Company
Waltham, MA

Prepared for the Anesthesia Patient Safety Foundation and
  supported by grants from Hewlett Packard Company,
  Ohmeda, and Puritan-Bennett.

Foreword by Ellison C. Pierce, Jr., M.D., President, Anesthesia
  Patient Safety Foundation

Butterworths
Boston   London   Singapore   Sydney   Toronto   Wellington

Every effort has been made to ensure that the drug dosage schedules,
descriptions of equipment, and diagnostic and therapeutic recommendations within this text are accurate and conform to standards
accepted at time of publication. However, as treatment recommendations vary in the light of continuing research and clinical experience, the reader is advised to verify drug dosage schedules and
diagnostic and therapeutic recommendations herein with information
found on product information sheets. This is especially true in cases
of new or infrequently used drugs.

Library of Congress Cataloging-in-Publication Data
Gravenstein, J. S.
  Capnography in clinical practice / Joachim S.
Gravenstein, David A. Paulus, and Thomas J. Hayes:
foreword by Ellison C. Pierce, Jr.
  p. cm.
  "Prepared for the Anesthesia Patient Safety Foundation."
  Includes index.
  ISBN 0-409-90135-0
  1. Capnography. I. Paulus, David A. II. Hayes,
Thomas J. III. Anesthesia Patient Safety Foundation.
IV. Title.
  [DNLM: 1. Anesthesia, General. 2. Carbon Dioxide—
analysis. 3. Monitoring, Physiologic—methods.
4. Respiratory Function Tests. WO 275 G775c]
RD82.G69 1988
617'.962—dc19
                                      88-14468

British Library Cataloguing in Publication Data
Gravenstein, Joachim S. (Joachim Stefan), 1925–
  Capnography in clinical practice
  1. Medicine Anaesthesia. Monitoring in applications of
capnography
  I. Title II. Paulus, David A. III. Hayes, Thomas J.
  617'.96
  ISBN 0-409-90135-0

Butterworth Publishers
80 Montvale Avenue
Stoneham, MA 02180

10 9 8 7 6 5 4 3 2 1

Printed in the United States of America

Contents

Foreword

The need for greater educational efforts in understanding capnography was recognized by the Anesthesia Patient Safety Foundation (APSF) shortly after its organization in the fall of 1985. The Foundation's Executive Committee decided to approach the problem by arranging for the production of a videotape and accompanying manual on the subject through the Committee on Education and Training.

Subsequently, the Hewlett Packard Company graciously provided funding and technical expertise for the filming of the videotape in Gainesville at the University of Florida. The proposed accompanying manual grew into this current volume. The Foundation is heavily indebted to Drs. Gravenstein and Paulus for their roles in bringing this undertaking to fruition. This educational endeavor clearly demonstrates the mission and purposes of the Foundation, which follow:

The mission of the Anesthesia Patient Safety Foundation is to assure that no patient shall be harmed by the effects of anesthesia.
The purposes of the Foundation are:

1. To foster investigations that will provide a better understanding of preventable anesthetic injuries.
2. To encourage programs that will reduce the number of anesthetic injuries.
3. To promote national and international communication of information about the causes and prevention of anesthetic injuries.

Ellison C. Pierce, Jr., M.D.
President
Anesthesia Patient Safety Foundation

Preface

For several decades capnography has been used in special cases; for example, neurosurgical operations that require fine adjustments in ventilation to attain particular arterial carbon dioxide concentrations. During the last few years anesthesiologists and intensivists have begun to extend the indication for capnography in routine anesthesia and monitoring ventilation in critically ill patients. Many clinicians now consider capnography a requisite for safe general anesthesia and proper ventilator management. Such wide acceptance was undoubtedly furthered by the discovery that monitoring carbon dioxide in the respired gas can quickly establish whether the trachea has been intubated successfully or whether, instead, the esophagus has been intubated by mistake, a dreadful cause of anesthetic disaster.

Clinicians familiar with capnography recognize many other obvious as well as subtle advantages of this monitoring technique. Capnography enables us to diagnose respiratory arrest and shunt, to assess—in conjunction with other measurements—pulmonary blood flow, and to suspect embolism and even cardiac arrest. We use capnography to adjust mechanical ventilators and locate incompetent valves in ventilatory or anesthetic circuitry, and to detect changes in alveolar dead space, decreases or increases in production of carbon dioxide, and disconnections of the patient from the mechanical ventilator—to name only some of the possibilities that enter into the differential diagnosis when capnography alerts the clinician to abnormal data.

Although this book covers much ground, it is not encyclopedic. We present in three parts what the clinician may want to learn about capnography. The first part deals with the clinical aspects of capnography; the second, the physiology of carbon dioxide as measured by capnography; and the third, the technology of capnography. Clinicians may want to study the first section, browse through the second, and consult the third for detailed technical explanations.

We had much help in preparing this book. The Anesthesia Patient Safety Foundation (APSF) encouraged us to proceed; the Hewlett Packard Company enabled us to employ an expert to review the technical literature. The Hewlett Packard Company also sponsored the production of a videotape on capnography that is available either through their company or the APSF. The videotape makes a useful educational companion to this book.

We wish to recognize colleagues who read early drafts of the book and offered many valuable suggestions; we are indebted to Drs. P.G. Boysen, N.

Gravenstein, and R.R. Kirby from the Department of Anesthesiology, and M. Jaeger from the Department of Physiology, all from the College of Medicine of the University of Florida, and to R.A. Parker, Ph.D., of Hewlett Packard. We owe special thanks to M.J. Banner, who not only read the text critically but was most helpful in setting up the demonstrations of the mechanical lung. We also thank G.Y. Nilsson of Hewlett Packard for preparing the illustrations in Part III. Finally, we thank Lynn Dirk, who patiently and expertly edited the entire text. A few stylistic excesses, however, are ours.

The careful reader may find mistakes in this book. If so, we gladly assume responsibility for them. Gladly, because could we write such a text without mistakes, we would have halos, and that would deny us many pleasures of this world.

J.S.G.
D.A.P.
T.J.H.

PART I

Clinical Perspectives on Capnography

Chapter 1

Carbon Dioxide and Monitoring

CARBON DIOXIDE TERMINOLOGY

First a word about words. *Capnograph* and *capnogram* hail from Greek: *capnos* (καπνός) "smoke" and *graphein* (γράφειν) "to write." In the context of clinical practice, the smoke can be thought of as rising from the fires of metabolism. A graphic plot of the concentrations of carbon dioxide as a function of time is called a capnogram, *gram* coming from *gramma* (γράμμα) "something written." The formulation of *capnometer* owes its existence to a custom dating back to the 17th century of adding the suffix *meter* (of mixed heritage) to denote an instrument for measuring. Concentrations of carbon dioxide, therefore, are depicted graphically as a capnogram, recorded by a capnograph, and measured by a capnometer. The practices of measuring and recording carbon dioxide are capnometry and capnography, respectively. Not all capnometers generate capnograms, but all capnographs are, or are a part of, capnometers.

Related terms are *hypercapnia* (also called hypercarbia), an abnormally high level of carbon dioxide, and *hypocapnia* (or *hypocarbia*), an abnormally low level of carbon dioxide. *Hypercapnia* and *hypocapnia* are understood (but semantically not specified) to relate to concentrations of carbon dioxide in blood, whether venous or arterial. These terms have led to confusion because hypocapnia, as measured in exhaled gas by capnometry, may fail to reflect concurrent hypercapnia in arterial or venous blood. Normal arterial values for carbon dioxide tension lie between 36 and 44 mm Hg.

GENERATING A CAPNOGRAM

There are two ways of presenting carbon dioxide concentrations in inhaled and exhaled gases. One way is to generate a capnogram that shows all changes in carbon dioxide concentrations throughout inspiration and expiration; this requires almost continuous measurement of carbon dioxide in the respired gas and almost continuous plotting of the measured values (Figures 1.1 and 1.2).

3

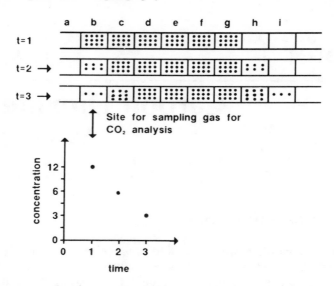

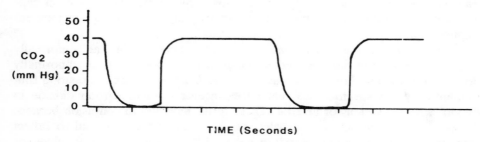

FIGURE 1.1   *Movement of carbon dioxide in a tube. Diagrammatic representation of how a capnogram is generated. At time t = 1, a tube consisting of segments **a** through **i** contains carbon dioxide in segments **b** through **g**. At time t = 2, half a segment of fresh gas is pushed into segment **a**, half of which is pushed into segment **b**, and so on. The process is repeated at time t = 3. Carbon dioxide concentration is analyzed in segment **b** at times t = 1, t = 2, and t = 3 and the data are plotted. Connecting the points of the plot with a line generates a capnogram.*

FIGURE 1.2   *A normal capnogram. On the ordinate, concentration is expressed as the partial pressure of carbon dioxide in mm Hg or torr but could also be presented in volume percent. On the abscissa, time is expressed in seconds. The partial pressure of gases can also be expressed in kPa. See inside back cover for conversion table from mm Hg to kPa.*

The other way is to rely on the capnometer to detect the highest and the lowest concentrations of carbon dioxide and to report these values as end-tidal and inspired minimal carbon dioxide concentrations, respectively. The nomenclature of the values reported, however, can be misleading. For several reasons, we should not speak of alveolar concentration of carbon dioxide when we are measuring the gas close to the patient's mouth, or even in the trachea. For instance, carbon dioxide concentrations probably vary among alveoli (see "Cardiogenic Oscillation" in Chapter 2); also, the highest concentration of carbon dioxide in the expired gas may not represent the alveolar or arterial concentration. We can refer to this highest value as peak concentration in the expired gas or, assuming that the peak will occur at the end of expiration, the end-tidal concentration.

An important distinction to remember with capnography is that the capnogram does not reflect gas flow. The last part of the capnogram (just before the plateau drops) is often not synonymous with the end of expiration. Therefore, the concentration of carbon dioxide measured at the end of the capnographic plateau may not be truly "end-tidal." After a healthy person takes a deep breath, the peak exhalation value of carbon dioxide may come within a few mm Hg of the arterial value.

Where to Sample Gas

The closer to the alveolus we sample gas, the more faithfully should the capnogram reflect what is in the alveolus and, hence, both in the pulmonary venous blood draining the lung and in the arterial blood. However, mucus and moisture in the upper airways create technical problems in placing a sampling catheter into the trachea and, thus, militate against intratracheal sampling. Another argument against intratracheal sampling, especially in a tracheally intubated patient, is the possibility of a ventilator disconnection. When a patient can breathe spontaneously, a capnogram from a sample of intratracheal gas does not reveal a disconnection of ventilator from patient (or at least not as rapidly) as would a capnogram of gas sampled from the breathing circuit itself. Many disconnections occur between endotracheal tube and Y connector, *i.e.*, between capnometer sampling site and endotracheal tube, in which case a disconnection will be discovered at once. In this book, unless otherwise stated, we will assume that the gas used for capnographic analysis is gas that was close to the patient's mouth but not actually in the patient.

THE VALUE OF A WAVEFORM

There is much to be learned on inspection of the capnogram. If algorithms could be designed that could reliably distinguish artifacts from clinical abnormalities in capnograms, and if the algorithm could reliably interpret the different patterns of capnographic waveforms, inspection of the capnogram would not be necessary. Until such algorithms are clinically tested and found reliable, however, we advise inspection of capnograms rather than of just peak exhaled and inhaled values reported digitally by a capnometer that does not have a capnograph. Errors in diagnosis can result when the capnogram is not or cannot be inspected (Figure 1.3).

Finally, plotting capnograms on slowly moving paper (or slowly advancing plots on an electronic display) enables the clinician to recognize trends of rising or falling concentrations of carbon dioxide in the inhaled and the exhaled gas. It is difficult (or impossible) to discern such trends in rows of numbers compared with a capnographic plot (Figure 1.4).

CAPNOGRAPHIC ANALYZERS

There are two types of capnographs: mainstream and sidestream (Figures 1.5 and 1.6). Both types sample gas close to the patient's mouth. Many different models are commercially available, and many are suitable and reliable. A detailed discussion of sampling technology and instruments can be found in Part III. Here we present a brief summary of mainstream and sidestream analyzers.

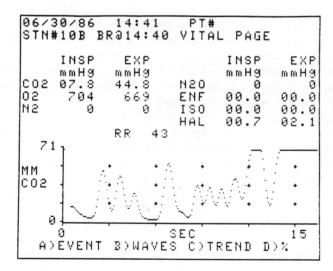

FIGURE 1.3   *Capnogram versus capnometric values. Page from a mass spectrometer with a reasonably sophisticated algorithm that reported the wrong end-tidal carbon dioxide concentration in a child in respiratory distress. The digital data show an expired value for carbon dioxide of 44.8 mm Hg; the true end-tidal value, however, was greater than 70 mm Hg. The error would not have been detected had the clinician not inspected the capnogram.*

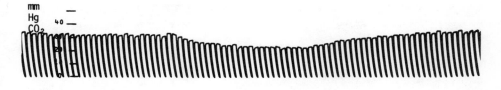

|←—1 min—→|

FIGURE 1.4 *Trends in capnograms. This capnogram shows a trend of slow decrease in peak expiratory carbon dioxide (CO_2) from about 34 to a low of 22 mm Hg, and then an increase to 35 mm Hg. Inspiratory values remained normal. This trend is compatible with a brief shower of air emboli in a patient undergoing a posterior fossa craniectomy in the sitting position.*

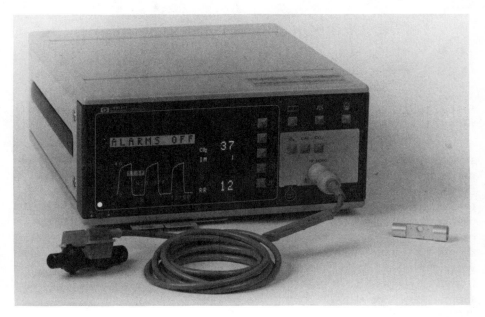

FIGURE 1.5 *A modern mainstream capnograph. A mainstream capnograph (Hewlett Packard) with two cuvettes: one for adults, with a volume of 15 ml, and one for neonates and babies (on the right), with a volume of 2 ml.*

Mainstream Analyzers

The mainstream analyzer generates a capnogram practically instantaneously because the gas is analyzed as it passes through the cuvette. This generates brisk capnograms, *i.e.*, the capnogram displays carbon dioxide levels in the

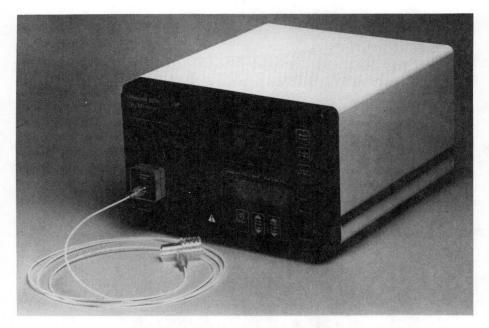

FIGURE 1.6   *A modern sidestream capnograph. A sidestream capnograph (Ohmeda) with a sampling connector.*

sampled gas with minimal delay because the response of the analyzer is not preceded by the time necessary for transport of gas from the sample port to the analyzer. With mainstream analyzers, a delay in response must be attributed to the analyzer itself. A disadvantage of some mainstream analyzers is the weight of the sensor and sampling cuvette, which contain essential components of the capnometer. Because the sensor itself is a sophisticated instrument, it should be treated with some deference; replacements are expensive. The volume of the cuvette adds dead space to the system. When gas is to be sampled from the hypopharynx or nostril, as is sometimes necessary in patients breathing spontaneously, an aspirating pump can pull the gas through the cuvette.

Sidestream Analyzers

The sidestream analyzer offers the advantage that gas is sampled close to the patient's mouth with the help of an inexpensive, lightweight connector (Figure 1.6). A disadvantage is that analysis is delayed because gas is routed through a capillary to the capnometer. The delay due to the transit time depends on the length and the diameter of the capillary and the rate at which the gas is aspirated (usually from 50 to 250 ml/min). The inherent response time of the capnometer itself causes a slight additional delay.

The gas sample can be viewed as a plug that moves through the tubing; the front and back of this plug are subject to mixing with other gas in the tube. Therefore, the shorter the transit time through the tube, the less mixing that occurs and the more representative the capnogram. Therefore, slow rates of flow, long capillaries with large lumen, or both will slur the upstroke and the downstroke of the capnogram (Figure 1.7). (See Part III.)

Because the sidestream analyzer removes gas from the patient's breathing circuit, two difficulties arise. One is what to do with the aspirated gas after it has been sampled. Gas that contains anesthetic agents should not be vented into the room. Returning the gas to the patient, however, through the breathing system without being able to clean and perhaps even sterilize the conduits through which the gas travels could expose the patient to whatever infectious agents the previous patient had exhaled into the conduits. It is best to scavenge the aspirated gas. Even though this is not difficult, it constitutes an encumbrance because the scavenging system itself introduces two possible difficulties. A

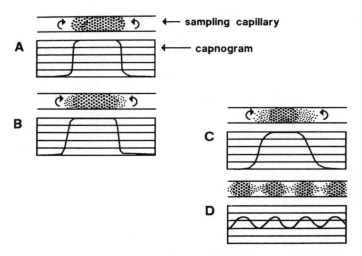

FIGURE 1.7 *The capnograph gas sample. A plug of carbon dioxide gas (stippled area) in a sampling capillary. Below the sampling capillary is the capnogram that would result were this plug to reach a carbon dioxide analyzer. As long as the front and back of the plug are well defined (as in A), the resultant capnogram will have a sharp upstroke and downstroke. As the boundaries of the plug become diffuse, the capnogram grows more and more slurred (B and C). In D several carbon dioxide plugs, as would occur during rapid ventilation with small tidal volumes, follow each other, all resulting in capnographic waves with poorly defined upstrokes and downstrokes, which creates an undulating appearance. Peak values of neither expired nor inspired carbon dioxide can be deduced from the capnogram in D. In order to obtain representative end-tidal values, the rapid ventilation has to be interrupted with a couple of slow, deep breaths, which allows the capnogram to display true inspiratory and end-tidal values.*

scavenging system may resist gas flow and thereby affect the pressure in the analyzing chamber, or the scavenger may generate a vacuum and thereby affect the sampling flow of the capnograph. Either possibility can cause errors; in order to prevent these errors, the capnograph should be calibrated with the scavenging system incorporated.

In closed anesthesia systems (only enough gas is added to the anesthesia breathing circuit to satisfy the requirement for oxygen and anesthesia and no excess gas needs to be vented), the capnometric gas sample constitutes a significant portion of fresh gas that must be restored to the system. Many patients consume no more than 200 ml/min of oxygen, which may be about as much as the capnometer also aspirates. In selecting the proper rate of gas flow in a closed system, the capnographic gas consumption and the physiologic gas requirement complicate the calculation of the patient's anesthetic uptake, even if one is fortunate enough to have an analyzer with which to measure anesthetic gas concentrations in the inhaled and exhaled gas mixtures.

Chapter 2

The Capnogram

THE NORMAL CAPNOGRAM

The normal capnogram resembles the outline of a snake that has just swallowed an elephant (with apologies to Antoine de Saint-Exupéry). The snake, however, is hiding in sand, and only the part containing the elephant rises above the sand (Figure 2.1). Such a picture gives the impression that a capnogram is a simple thing. It is not; but a normal capnogram does have the outline of a snake that has eaten an elephant.

PHASES OF THE CAPNOGRAM

We distinguish four phases of a capnogram. Let us assume that the sampling port for carbon dioxide, or the capnometer cuvette, is properly positioned close to the mouth of the patient or at the end of the endotracheal tube. The first phase is the flat part of the capnogram, during inspiration. We shall have more to say about this phase later.

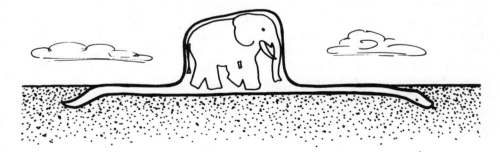

FIGURE 2.1 *The "capnophant." The normal capnogram has the outline of an elephant swallowed by a snake hiding under sand. (Image suggested from a drawing by the Little Prince—without his knowledge, but certainly his blessing if he could be found.)*

The second phase of the capnogram is the ascending part (we are approaching the elephant from behind). This corresponds to the appearance of carbon dioxide during exhalation. Exhalation actually begins a little before Phase II because the first gas to appear under the sampling port during exhalation is the gas that was last inhaled into the conducting airways (anatomic dead space); this gas has not been subjected to gas exchange and, thus, is essentially free of carbon dioxide. Soon, however, the first carbon dioxide appears and the capnogram begins an upstroke.

The third phase is marked by a plateau of the capnogram (the back of the elephant). Normally, this plateau remains nearly constant until the next inspiration sweeps away the carbon dioxide, but constancy of the capnogram plateau does not mean constant flow. Exhalation and a slightly rising carbon dioxide concentration may coexist if there is no uneven venting of different parts of the lungs. Then exhalation comes to an end, and in many instances a respiratory pause supervenes. During this time gas does not flow and the last carbon dioxide is deposited at the sampling site. As long as that pertains, the plateau persists. In patients in whom exhalation progresses abnormally slowly (*e.g.,* in asthmatics) expiratory gas flow continues until the capnographic curve begins its downslope. Sidestream analyzers may aspirate fresh gas, and the plateau can then slope downward until the next inspiration sweeps away the last carbon dioxide.

The fourth phase is marked by the downward direction of the capnogram (sliding down the forehead and trunk of the elephant). This downstroke corresponds to the fresh gas that passes the sampling port during inspiration. Because inspiration starts well before the capnogram returns to baseline, we list the first phase of the capnogram last.

During the first phase the capnogram holds steady at zero (as long as the snake holds still). For part of the first phase, inspiration is in progress; after a brief pause expiration begins. Not until the capnograph begins to sense the first carbon dioxide can we detect this change of direction in flow.

To demonstrate these four phases of the capnogram and their relationship to inhaled and exhaled flow and airway presure, we arranged to collect capnograms generated simultaneously by a mainstream and a sidestream analyzer attached to a mechanical lung into which we infused carbon dioxide. The lung was attached to a ventilator that was set at a respiratory rate of 10 breaths/min (Figure 2.2). Changes in pressure and flow slightly preceded the deflection in the mainstream capnogram (Figure 2.3). The sidestream analyzer was out of phase by about 3 seconds because of the delay introduced by transport of the gas sample through the capillary to the analyzer.

THE ABNORMAL CAPNOGRAM

Abnormalities in a capnogram are identified by the phase in which they appear.

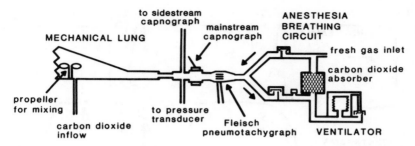

FIGURE 2.2   *Equipment configuration to demonstrate the relationships between the capnogram and the pressure, flow, and volume of gas. Carbon dioxide, 300 ml/ min, was infused into a mechanical lung in which a fan stirred the gas. The lung was connected to an anesthesia circle system with a ventilator and both a mainstream and a sidestream capnograph attached.*

Phase II: The Slanted Upstroke

A slow rate of sampling significantly prolongs the interval between when the breath occurs and when the capnogram is inscribed (Figure 2.4). The shape of the capnogram also is affected by a slow rate of sampling. With slow sampling, the upstroke becomes slanted. Also, during inspiration the capnogram may not have time to reach zero (compared with the capnogram of the mainstream analyzer). In the example shown in Figure 2.4, the capnogram falsely shows a carbon dioxide tension of about 7 mm Hg during inspiration. With the slower sampling rate the plateau becomes rounded.

If a slanted upstroke cannot be explained on the basis of delayed response of equipment, expiratory time may be prolonged (carbon dioxide is emerging too slowly from the lungs, for instance, because of obstruction). The capnogram does not reflect flow, only concentration of carbon dioxide. As long as the capnogram is recording changes, there must be some gas flow to cause concentration to fluctuate at the sensor, but we cannot tell how much. Flow may be normal, but the concentration of carbon dioxide in the exhaled gas rises over time as different segments of the lungs empty sequentially. If the instrument or sampling rate cannot be blamed for a slant in Phase II, uneven emptying of the lungs is the most likely cause. A capnogram in which Phase II becomes severely slanted and shortened and continues into Phase III typifies chronic obstructive lung disease and asthma.

Phase III: The Plateau

Abnormally High Plateau

Normal values for peak expiratory carbon dioxide partial pressure lie between 36 and 44 mm Hg. A number of physiologic events can cause the level of

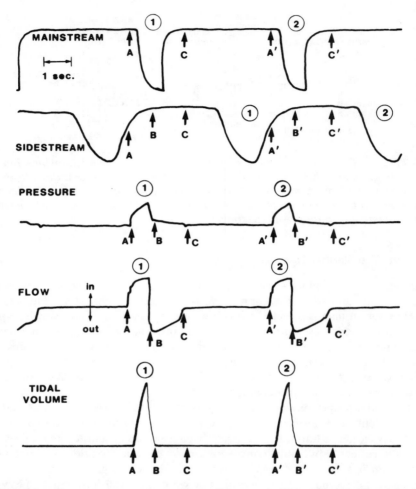

FIGURE 2.3   *Capnograms and pressure, flow, and tidal volume. Data obtained experimentally (Figure 2.2) are from a Hewlett Packard mainstream capnograph, a Datascope sidestream capnograph, a pressure transducer (upstroke = increased pressure), and a Fleisch pneumotachygraph (for flow, upstroke = inspiration), and inspiratory tidal volume. The curves were recorded by a Grass polygraph, which records in a circular path. The arrows point to identical times but are not perfectly aligned because of the way traces are recorded. For breath 1, observe that pressure, flow, and volume are recorded nearly simultaneously at A; the capnogram of the mainstream analyzer responds in less than 0.5 second. B indicates the moment of flow reversal (from inspiration to expiration). At C all flow ceases, but the mainstream capnogram registers carbon dioxide that remains under the sensor. Thus, capnographic evidence of carbon dioxide is indicated even though there is no gas flow. For breath 2 (A') gas begins to flow again and the cycle repeats. The capnogram of the sidestream analyzer is almost one full breath out of phase. It shows deflections from previous expirations at A and A'.*

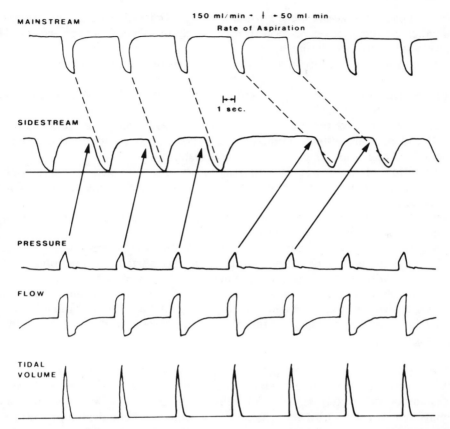

FIGURE 2.4   *The effect of rate of sampling flow on sidestream analyzers. Sampling at a flow rate of 150 ml/min with an experimental model (Figures 2.2 and 2.3), a capnogram from a sidestream analyzer indicates almost identical data as the capnogram of the mainstream analyzer (the inspired values are slightly elevated on the sidestream capnogram). However, when the sampling rate is reduced to 50 ml/min, the sidestream capnograph does not have time to return to baseline before the next breath begins. Here it falsely reports carbon dioxide at 7 mm Hg during Phase IV. With fast sampling the respiratory pause and, hence, the plateau phase are long enough for the slower sidestream analyzer to reach its full response. Therefore, in the examples shown here, peak expired values of sidestream and mainstream capnograms are similar for the first three breaths. Slow sampling with a sidestream analyzer when respiratory rate is high can result in erroneous values during inspiration and expiration.*

carbon dioxide to exceed these normal averages. For example, during normal, unmedicated, deep sleep, carbon dioxide levels in exhaled air can exceed 44 mm Hg as ventilation diminishes.

Clinically, end-tidal carbon dioxide can be increased in a variety of ways:

- increased carbon dioxide production, such as with malignant hyperpyrexia, fever, or excitement;
- depressed respiratory center, such as with narcotics, anesthetics, other central nervous system depressants, or toxic agents or acquired or inborn diseases that affect the central nervous system;
- inhibition of nerve impulses to respiratory muscles, such as with polio-myelitis, Guillain-Barré syndrome, or many other afflictions of the nervous system;
- blockade of the neuromuscular junction, such as with neuromuscular blocking drugs or myasthenia gravis;
- weakened respiratory muscles, such as with muscular dystrophies;
- lung dysfunction, such as with asthma, chronic obstructive pulmonary disease, or with respiratory distress syndromes during thoracotomy;
- obstructed airways, such as with papillomatosis, tumors internal or external to the airways, burns, congenital narrowing of the airways, inflammatory swelling including croup or diphtheria, or allergic swelling as from bee stings.

All the diseases and conditions on this list are merely examples and do not represent an exhaustive recitation of possible causes. When any of these problems occur in conjunction with another, a mild to moderate respiratory impairment can soon turn into disaster. Inadequate mechanical ventilation in the operating room is all too common. The postanesthesia care unit is an area fraught with serious hazards that are well recognized[1] and that stem from inadequate spontaneous ventilation of patients still under the influence of anesthetics, narcotics, and muscle relaxants as well as the effects of the operation. These effects, often in concert with constricting bandages, can conspire to increase exhaled and arterial carbon dioxide levels and eventually can cause respiratory arrest. It is often forgotten that, even in healthy volunteers, the combination of clinical doses of a narcotic analgesic drug and a small dose of a neuromuscular blocking drug potentiate each other's inhibiting effect on ventilation.[2]

When the peak expiratory values are elevated above a normal level and stay there for several minutes (Figure 2.5), retention of carbon dioxide in blood is certain. Patients with chronic diseases affecting pulmonary gas exchange are accustomed to (and to a degree compensate for) elevated carbon dioxide concentrations in their blood. It may be impossible (and at times unwise) to alter such increased levels of carbon dioxide. However, when the end-tidal carbon dioxide levels increase from a normal baseline, the clinician, remembering that hypoventilation with hypercapnia is associated with hypoxia when

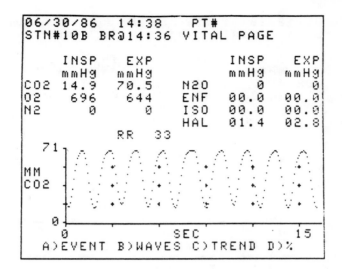

```
06/30/86   14:38    PT#
STN#10B  BR@14:36  VITAL PAGE

       INSP     EXP            INSP     EXP
       mmHg     mmHg           mmHg     mmHg
CO2    14.9     70.5    N20       0        0
O2      696      644    ENF     00.0     00.0
N2        0        0    ISO     00.0     00.0
                       HAL     01.4     02.8
                RR   33
   71
MM
CO2

    0
       0            SEC              15
     A)EVENT  B)WAVES  C)TREND  D)%
```

FIGURE 2.5.   *Capnogram showing hypoventilation. Expiratory and inspiratory carbon dioxide levels were grossly elevated in this patient, a child being improperly mechanically ventilated with a Bain circuit. Increasing fresh gas flow and continuing mechanical ventilation reduced both inspiratory and expiratory carbon dioxide values to normal.*

the patient is breathing room air, must make a diagnosis (is it the patient or the equipment?) and proceed to correct the problem.

Transient Occurrences of This Abnormality.   When establishing a systemic-to-pulmonary artery shunt, the surgeon, while making the anastomosis, clamps the pulmonary artery of one lung. Once this clamp is released, end-tidal carbon dioxide tension increases as the lung is reperfused. Similarly, release of tourniquets on ischemic limbs or release of aortic clamps can also briefly increase end-tidal carbon dioxide. Intravenous administration of bicarbonate or insufflation of carbon dioxide, for instance into the peritoneal cavity during laparoscopy, also elevates the carbon dioxide in blood and subsequently the alveolar carbon dioxide concentration. These transient increases in exhaled carbon dioxide occur only when there is a constant rate of ventilation. When patients breathe into artificial systems or are dependent on mechanical ventilation, defects in the mechanical system also can elevate end-exhaled carbon dioxide levels, but this is a factor related to dead space.

Abnormally Low Plateau

When the plateau hovers at levels less than 36 mm Hg (Figure 2.6) in a patient dependent on mechanical ventilation, a number of clinical considerations should arise. Are the patient's lungs hyperventilated? Check the ventilator settings or, even better, use a spirometer on the expiratory limb of the breathing

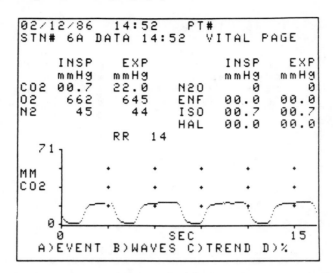

FIGURE 2.6 *Capnogram showing hyperventilation. The expiratory carbon dioxide levels in this patient were abnormally low, secondary to excessive mechanical ventilation.*

system.* A minute volume of 100 to 120 ml/kg body weight or tidal volume of 10 to 12 ml/kg and a respiratory rate of about 10 breaths/min should restore proper gas values. Many factors can modify the patient's ventilatory requirements (see Part II). If hyperventilation is not causing low carbon dioxide levels in exhaled gas, consider decreased carbon dioxide production (low temperature?), decreased delivery of carbon dioxide to the lungs (embolism or low cardiac output?), or an improper setting of the ventilator (tidal volume too small to bring alveolar gas to the fore?). Also, mechanical artifacts can be deceptive by showing that the patient's lungs are hyperventilated when, in reality, the sidestream analyzer is aspirating room air, which dilutes the exhaled gas, through a crack in the sampling capillary or an ill-fitting connector.

A low level of end-tidal carbon dioxide can coexist with a high level of arterial carbon dioxide. Ventilation of unperfused segments of the lung (not common during anesthesia) may cause a large gradient from arterial (high) to alveolar (low) carbon dioxide tension.

In summary, an abnormally low plateau in the capnogram often reflects hyperventilation, but the arterial carbon dioxide tension may be normal or

---

*The excursion of the bellows on the anesthesia ventilator indicates only the level of tidal volume that the ventilator delivers; the anesthesia machine, however, delivers an additional volume of fresh gas that can substantially affect tidal volume. Assume the tidal volume of the respirator is set at 800 ml, inspiratory-to-expiratory time (I:E) at 1:2, and rate at 10 breaths/min. The minute volume of the respirator will be 8000 ml. Assume now that the fresh gas flow is 5 L/min. Because inhalation constitutes 20 seconds of every minute (I:E = 1:2), 33% of 5 L (20 seconds of every minute), or 1.6 L, will be added to the 8-L minute volume indicated by the ventilator.

even higher than normal. When in doubt, arterial blood should be analyzed for carbon dioxide and oxygen.

The Irregular Plateau

Bumps and Dips.   Ordinarily, the capnogram plateau runs horizontally, or almost so. Bumps and dips in the plateau can be either artifactual or physiologic. An artifactual bump can be caused by pushing on the chest of an anesthetized patient, which causes a little gas to move in and out of the lungs, which, in turn, causes the plateau to undulate (Figure 2.7). Such artifacts are common during anesthesia and surgical procedures.

If no one has pushed down on the patient's chest, a dip indicates a spontaneous breath by a patient who is not paralyzed and is undergoing mechanical ventilation (Figure 2.8). The first breath initiated by a respiratory center that has been previously quiescent is typically a breath of small tidal volume, a breathlet, too small to remove all the carbon dioxide from the sampling site of the capnograph; thus, the capnogram does not return to baseline. Such a breathlet indicates that the respiratory center is being stimu-

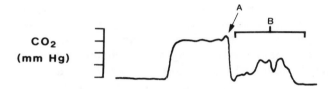

FIGURE 2.7   *Capnogram with an artifact in the plateau (Phase III). This patient was anesthetized and dependent on mechanical ventilation. Intraoperatively, the surgeon leaned on the patient's chest, which resulted first in a bump in the plateau of the capnogram (A) and then in irregular fluctuations in the inspiratory phase of the capnogram (B). The bump (A) signifies that mechanical ventilation in this anesthetized patient did not bring forth the highest concentration of carbon dioxide in the patient's lungs. Thus, the capnogram, even though it had a well-sustained plateau, did not register alveolar carbon dioxide levels.*

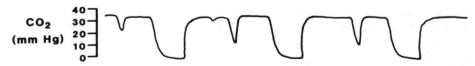

FIGURE 2.8   *Capnogram showing a breathlet in the plateau (Phase III). This capnogram shows a patient making inspiratory efforts during mechanical ventilation, but the capnogram cannot reveal the circumstances of the inspiratory effort. Only examination of the patient and analysis of all clinical factors can guide the clinician in deciding to adjust the ventilator, give drugs, or initiate other maneuvers. The patient's minute ventilation, level of anesthesia, degree of muscle relaxation, and metabolic state and the impact of external stimuli require consideration.*

lated by carbon dioxide, decreased pH, or a somatic stimulus such as pain. This breathlet prompts the clinician to decide whether therapeutic adjustments are required. If the patient normally commands full muscle power and has a fully responsive respiratory center, the breathlet may simply be a first, small, spontaneous inspiration such as would occur at the end of anesthesia, for instance. Another possibility is that the patient's lungs may have been hyperventilated and now carbon dioxide concentrations are permitted to rise slowly. In these situations each successive breath will be larger; soon the patient will breathe normally, and the clinician can simply be reassured that all is well. In the patient in full control of muscle power, a dip in the plateau may be acceptable as long as the patient does not fight the ventilator or, during anesthesia, as long as the extra breathlet is not a gasp of pain. In contrast, in paralyzed patients whose lungs are of necessity being mechanically ventilated, a dip may signify hypoventilation—that arterial carbon dioxide levels are too high. With deep paralysis respiratory muscles cannot respond. If paralysis is incomplete, very strong stimuli may overpower the weakness and cause small inspiratory efforts. A dip will appear in the plateau of the capnogram (Figure 2.8). Even more worrisome, a severely hypoxic patient may attempt to overcome near paralysis to suck in air.

Whether the dip in the plateau of the capnogram indicates the first, gentle effort to breathe spontaneously or desperate gasps for air must be deduced from physical signs. The first breathlet of a patient in full respiratory command and returning to spontaneous breathing is a smooth and coordinated inspiration; no motion can be detected in the patient's neck or in the larynx, and chest and abdomen rise almost imperceptibly. This is in stark contrast to the first breath of a patient still largely paralyzed. Because the normal innervation of the respiratory muscles fails to effect gas exchange, the respiratory center sends strong impulses to the diaphragm until finally it contracts enough to generate a breathlet, but the contraction is jerky, almost spastic, which with inspiration yanks the lungs and airways downward and also the larynx—the dreaded tracheal tug. If matters persist unchecked, auxiliary muscles are recruited and then, in an ominous progression, the floor of the mouth, the nares, and finally tongue and lips twitch with every inspiration—the picture of agonal breathing. During these frantic attempts to draw in air, the upper chest may fall as the abdomen rises. A similar picture is observed in patients with obstructed airways or any other condition in which normal innervation of the respiratory muscles does not effect normal gas exchange.

The dip in the plateau of the capnogram, therefore, requires a careful analysis that cannot be limited to inspection of the capnogram but must include the patient's status and the pattern of ventilation accompanying the dip. To refer to such dips as "curare clefts" may mislead the clinician into thinking that more muscle relaxant is needed. More neuromuscular blockade may indeed be called for but should be instituted only after a careful analysis of underlying mechanisms. More often than not, more muscle blockade is not needed;

instead, more anesthesia or more ventilation is required. At the end of anesthesia and after complete reversal of neuromuscular blockade, a dip generated by an effortless breathlet is a welcome sign that the patient is ready to assume spontaneous ventilation and the clinician can gradually discontinue mechanical ventilation. In anesthesia, if relying heavily on narcotics, it is vital to remember that these drugs are respiratory depressants; they may delay the first breathlets until carbon dioxide levels become markedly elevated.

Unevenness.   Sequential rather than simultaneous emptying of the two lungs, *i.e.*, one lung expelling gas later than the other, causes a wavering plateau (Figure 2.9).

The Slanted Plateau

A common capnographic feature typical of patients with asthma or chronic obstructive lung disease of different causes is the slanted plateau (Figure 2.10). The conditions indicated by a slanted plateau resemble uneven or sequential emptying of the two lungs; however, instead of two discrete segments of the lungs emptying out of sequence, uneven emptying occurs among many segments of the lung. Even if the plateau is slanted, however, as long as it rises, the patient continues to exhale. With slow exhalation, inhalation may come before the expired phase has run its course. So-called end-tidal values of carbon dioxide tension (PCO_2) may be well below alveolar PCO_2 and arterial PCO_2.

The Plateau and Various Leaks

During mechanical ventilation of a patient's lungs, a leak between the sampling capillary and the capnometer can cause a prominent peak in the plateau of the capnogram of a sidestream analyzer. The plateau itself will be reduced proportionally to the size of the leak. The plateau is reduced because the capnometer aspirates room air, together with exhaled gas. The peak, coming at the end of the plateau, reflects the wave of positive pressure and the beginning of inspiration that cancels the negative pressure that first caused room air to be aspirated. The size of the leak will influence the height of the plateau, while the amount of peak inspiratory pressure will influence the size of the peak, and thus how close the peak will come to reflecting true end-tidal values.[3]

A leak around the cuff of the endotracheal tube shortens the plateau and sometimes forces the plateau to slope downward (sliding down the trunk of the elephant). This happens when exhaled gas escapes through the leak around the cuff.

Finally, a strong negative phase of the ventilator can exacerbate the aspiration of room air through a leak in the sampling capillary of a sidestream analyzer. Thus, a dip in the plateau is caused.

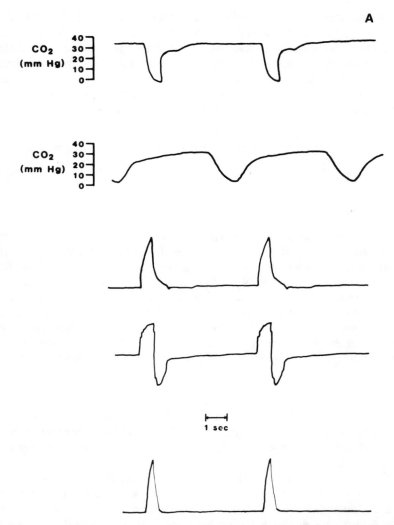

FIGURE 2.9   *Capnogram showing uneven emptying of the lungs. A mechanical lung (Figure 2.3) with two bellows was connected to a trachea via two mainstem bronchi. (A) Tracings (from top to bottom) are from a mainstream capnograph, a sidestream capnograph, a pressure transducer, a pneumotachygraph (for flow and tidal volume). For one lung, compliance was set at 0.02 L/cm H_2O and bronchial resistance at 2.5 cm H_2O/L/sec, and for the other lung 0.05 L/cm H_2O and 55 cm H_2O/L/sec, respectively. During ventilation the mainstream capnogram (top tracing) has a step increase in the plateau, which corresponds to one lung emptying before the other. The sidestream capnogram (second tracing from top) has a sloped plateau. The same type*

B

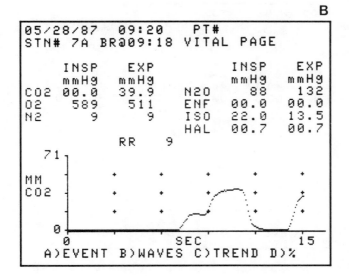

C

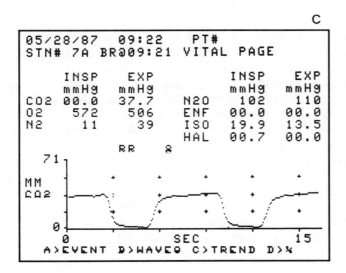

of capnogram was obtained from a patient under general anesthesia whose lungs emptied unevenly (B). After the trachea was suctioned (C), the capnogram returned to normal. We presume that suctioning removed a mucus plug that had partially occluded one lung.

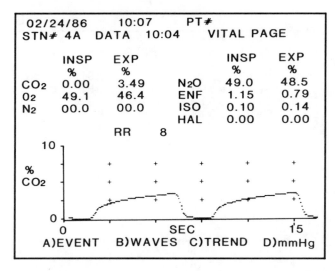

FIGURE 2.10   *Capnogram from a patient with severe obstructive lung disease.*

Phase IV: The Slanted Downstroke

Under ordinary circumstances during Phase IV the capnogram returns briskly to baseline as fresh gas replaces carbon dioxide at the sampling site. If this phase proceeds slowly (Figure 2.11), either inspiration is abnormally slow (unlikely because only very little gas is needed to replace the small volume of end-exhaled gas aspirated into the sampling site) or there was carbon dioxide in the inhaled gas, as may occur when the Bain system is used or when the inspiratory valve of a circle system is malfunctioning (Figure 2.11B).

Finally, independent of ventilation, fresh gas can dilute the gas sampled from the previous breath. This is often the case with sidestream analyzers, which aspirate gas from the connector attached to the patient's tracheal tube. As the end-tidal gas is aspirated, fresh gas flows in from the breathing system; this will gradually dilute the remaining carbon dioxide from the previous breath (Figure 2.11A). Such dilution may unmask cardiogenic oscillation in Phase IV of the capnogram (see "Cardiogenic Oscillation").

Phase I: The Abnormal Baseline

During mechanical ventilation, a capnogram that registers carbon dioxide during inspiration focuses attention on the patient or the system. If the surgeon leans on the patient's chest, which imposes external chest compression, the capnogram will reflect that (Figure 2.12). When the capnogram fails to return to baseline during inspiration and this is not explained by a slow capnographic

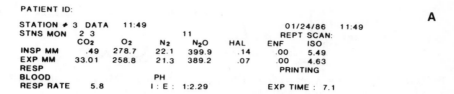

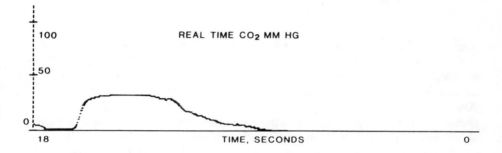

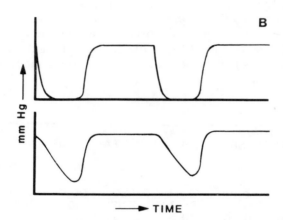

FIGURE 2.11 *Capnogram with abnormally prolonged downstroke (Phase IV). (A) A slant in the downstroke of a capnogram can be attributed to fresh gas pulled into the sampling site of a sidestream analyzer before the next breath removes the end-tidal gas of the previous sample. A sloped downstroke is more common with slow ventilation, which leaves much time for the continuous suction of the sidestream analyzer to aspirate fresh gas. (B) An incompetent inspiratory valve in a circle system can also cause the downstroke to be slanted. Compare a normal capnogram (upper tracing) and a capnogram with incompetent inspiratory unidirectional valve (lower tracing).*

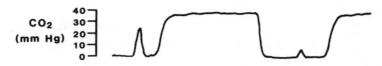

FIGURE 2.12   *Capnogram with an artifact in the baseline (Phase I). The capnogram shows a whiff of carbon dioxide that was raised from the depth of the patient's lungs when a tired surgeon leaned briefly on the patient's chest.*

response, then there must be some carbon dioxide in the inspired gas. A common reason for this is an exhausted carbon dioxide absorber, which fails to remove all the carbon dioxide. (Remember that the color indicator of many carbon dioxide absorbers does not reliably betray exhaustion of the absorber!) Also, with an improperly packed carbon dioxide absorber, gas may find a channel through the absorber and, thus, not all carbon dioxide would be absorbed. Even with a fresh, well-packed absorber, baseline carbon dioxide can be elevated during inspiration if the valves in the circle system malfunction. In valveless systems (*e.g.*, the Bain system), inadequate fresh gas flow also leads to rebreathing and the appearance of carbon dioxide in the inspired gas.

In spontaneously breathing patients abnormal respiratory patterns generate irregular capnograms (Figure 2.13). Although such irregularities are reflected in the capnogram, it is not the best means of diagnosing them. The capnogram is a poor mirror of flow.

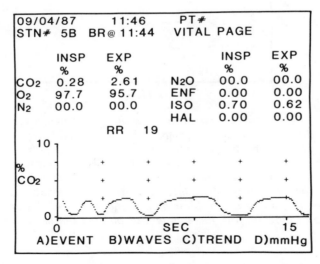

FIGURE 2.13   *Capnogram showing uneven and irregular ventilation. This may occur with a spontaneously breathing patient for a variety of reasons. Here, a conscious patient was distracted and, therefore, breathed unevenly and irregularly.*

CARDIOGENIC OSCILLATION

Undulations in the capnogram that are synchronous with cardiac contractions are called cardiogenic oscillations (Figure 2.14). The effect, which has been described many times,[4,5] is synchronous with changes in pulmonary blood volume. During systole, when contraction of the right heart fills the pulmonary vascular system, a small volume of gas is expelled from the lungs. During diastole, as blood drains from the pulmonary vascular system into the atrium and fills the ventricle, the heart generates a small inspiratory movement which, according to Arieli,[6] mainly affects the terminal bronchi of the lung. Capnograms from patients suffering severe emphysema tend not to register cardiogenic oscillations.

In patients paralyzed and dependent on mechanical ventilation, during the respiratory pause inspiratory and expiratory valves of the breathing system often open in sequence and in harmony with cardiac activity, which indicates that small volumes of gas are moving in and out of the lungs. A sensitive pneumotachygraph can record these small fluctuations in gas in the absence of ventilation; carbon dioxide at the sampling site is pushed slightly back and forth with each heartbeat. In many patients this does not produce cardiogenic oscillation in the capnogram. However, if at the same time a sidestream analyzer aspirates enough fresh gas, cardiogenic oscillations on the capnogram are likely.

In an experiment with a healthy male subject (Figure 2.15), ventricular

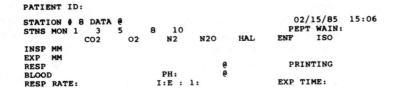

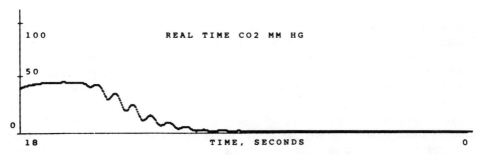

FIGURE 2.14 *Capnogram with cardiogenic oscillation. The effect is pronounced in this capnogram, which was generated with a sidestream analyzer (mass spectrometer).*

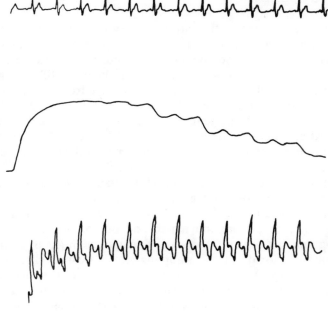

FIGURE 2.15   *Simultaneous electrocardiogram and capnogram with cardiogenic oscillations and pneumotachygram. Cardiogenic oscillations in this capnogram (middle) were generated from a healthy volunteer who breathed into a mouthpiece, to which a pneumotachygraph (set at high sensitivity) and sidestream capnograph sampling connector were attached. An electrocardiogram (top tracing) was recorded simultaneously. Oscillations appeared on the capnogram only on the downslope (Phase IV). The oscillation occurred at the same rate as the heartbeat, but they were not synchronous because of the delayed response of the sidestream capnograph, 2 to 3 seconds after the pneumotachygram (see Figure 2.3). In order to generate a pneumotachygram, the subject kept his glottis open after an exhalation was completed.*

contraction was associated with an inspiratory flow rate of about 33 ml/sec. Cardiogenic inspiration lasted only a fraction of a second, the tidal volume of which amounted to about 8 ml. Larger volumes have been reported, and in some patients cardiogenic oscillation can contribute a small percentage to minute volume and to gas exchange and can help to stir the gases in the lung.

In some persons a catheter placed just above the carina will show large fluctuations of carbon dioxide synchronous with cardiac activity.[7] Such fluctuations in concentration of any gas in the lungs can be observed if it is not the only gas present. Because these fluctuations can be seen during breathholding or apnea (no gas removed from deep in the lungs), the oscillation must be caused by rhythmic changes in the concentration of the gas, in this case, carbon dioxide. Only regional ventilation/perfusion differences can explain such dif-

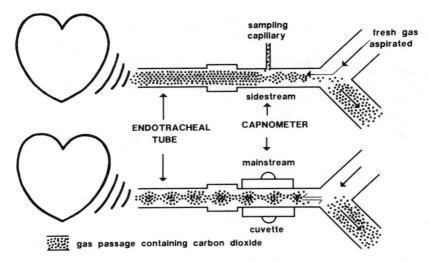

FIGURE 2.16   *Causes of cardiogenic oscillations in the capnogram. Cardiogenic oscillations affect capnograms in different ways. A sidestream analyzer removes carbon dioxide from the sampling site and simultaneously pulls in fresh gas; the effect of the heartbeat on the gas column—here assumed to be filled with the homogeneous carbon dioxide—registers on the capnogram because the carbon dioxide is mixed with fresh gas (top). This type of cardiogenic oscillation only occurs with sidestream analyzers just before inspiration. Cardiogenic oscillation, however, can also be observed in the tracheal tube (and at the mouth) when cardiac activity propels gas from different segments of the lungs when they empty unevenly and have ventilation-to-perfusion abnormalities of varying degrees (bottom). This type of cardiogenic oscillation would be reflected on capnograms from both sidestream and mainstream analyzers.*

ferences in concentration of carbon dioxide (or any other gas) between adjoining segments of the lung. Indeed, cardiogenic oscillations have been used to study ventilation and perfusion abnormalities in the lungs.[8]

Cardiogenic oscillations on the capnogram can be generated by the aspiration of fresh gas, even if there were no differences in carbon dioxide concentration in the lower airways (Figure 2.16, *top*). They can also be transmitted from deep in the lung (Figure 2.16, *bottom*).

REFERENCES

1. Wood MD: Monitoring equipment and loss reduction: An insurer's view, in Gravenstein JS, Holzer JF (eds): Safety and Cost Containment in Anesthesia. Boston, Butterworths, 1988, pp 47–54
2. Bellville JW, Cohen EN, Hamilton J: The interaction of morphine and *d*-tubocurarine on respiration and grip strength in man. Clin Pharmacol Ther 5:35–43, 1964

3. Zupan J, Martin M, Benumof J: End-tidal CO_2 excretion waveform and error with gas sampling line leak. Anesth Analg 67:579–581, 1988
4. Dahlstrom H, Murphy JP, Roos A: Cardiogenic oscillations in composition of expired gas. The "pneumocardiogram." J Appl Physiol 7:335–339, 1954
5. Fowler KT, Read J: Cardiac oscillations in expired gas tensions and regional pulmonary blood flow. J Appl Physiol 16:863–868, 1961
6. Arieli R: Cardiogenic oscillations in expired gas: Origin and mechanism. Respir Physiol 52:191–204, 1983
7. Nunn JF, Hill DW: Respiratory dead space and arterial to end-tidal CO_2 tension difference in anesthetized man. J Appl Physiol 15:383–389, 1960
8. Fowler KT, Read J: Cardiogenic oscillations as an index of pulmonary blood flow distribution. J Appl Physiol 18:233–243, 1963

Chapter 3

Dead Space

Dead space is simple and complex at the same time. It is a space through which gas must come and go without losing oxygen or gaining carbon dioxide in significant amounts. During exhalation, dead space fills with carbon dioxide-containing gas, which during inhalation is replaced by fresh gas drawn (or during mechanical ventilation pumped) into the lungs.

Increased dead space risks retention of carbon dioxide. Rebreathing is possible whenever the open, natural atmosphere from which we breathe air is restricted, for instance when a paper bag is placed over the head, surgical drapes cover the face, or when our lungs are ventilated through an artificial system. Such artificial systems consist of conduits with or without valves, may or may not include a carbon dioxide absorber, and may be used with or without a mechanical ventilator. All have the potential to add mechanical dead space to the physiologic dead space of the respiratory tract. It is therefore necessary to recognize abnormal dead space.

Total dead space, often called physiologic dead space, can be measured clinically. Part of the total dead space, called anatomic dead space, encloses the internal volume of the upper airways (nose, pharynx, trachea, and bronchi). When a tracheostomy tube or an endotracheal tube bypasses mouth and nose, anatomic dead space is reduced. Placing a mask over a patient's face and attaching a tube to the mask through which the patient must inhale and exhale enlarges the anatomic dead space by the volume of the mask and the tube, but we will not have increased dead space if we set aside the mask and simply inhale fresh (carbon dioxide-free) gas through one tube and exhale carbon dioxide-laden gas through another tube. The anesthesia circle systems in common use, therefore, do not add much dead space as long as the unidirectional valves (for inhalation and exhalation) are competent and the carbon dioxide absorber functions. The volume of the face-mask and the volume of the Y piece that connects the mask (or endotracheal tube) to the breathing tubes constitute the mechanical dead space. A so-called gooseneck extension between endotracheal tube and Y piece and a sampling cuvette for the capnograph also add to the mechanical dead space.

Although anatomic dead space is largely constant, one component of physiologic dead space can vary considerably, *i.e.*, alveolar dead space. Alveoli that are ventilated and perfused and that participate in gas exchange are not part of the dead space, but alveoli that are underperfused while ventilated do contribute to dead space.[1] Because variations in the ventilation-to-perfusion ratio are common, the alveolar dead space is thought of as variable. The total physiologic dead space, therefore, is also variable. (See Part II for more detail.) If the conduits do not change and if part of a ventilated lung is not perfused, the physiologic dead space increases by the gas volume of that part of the lung.

From the perspective of ventilation, dead space is defined as minute ventilation minus effective alveolar ventilation. For a single breath, the effective alveolar tidal volume is total tidal volume − dead space. The famous ratio of dead space to tidal volume (V_D/V_T) is calculated from the Enghoff equation (modified from the Bohr equation) as follows:

$$\frac{V_D}{V_T} = \frac{PaCO_2 - P\bar{E}CO_2}{PaCO_2}$$

where V_D is dead space, V_T is tidal volume, $PaCO_2$ is the partial pressure of carbon dioxide in arterial blood, and $P\bar{E}CO_2$ is the mean partial pressure of exhaled carbon dioxide in the total exhaled volume of gas after thorough mixing. To rearrange the formula and solve for dead space is easy:

$$V_D = \frac{PaCO_2 - P\bar{E}CO_2}{PaCO_2} \times V_T$$

Normally, exhaled gas is collected in a bag over 3 minutes and the $P\bar{E}CO_2$ is measured from the bag ($P\bar{E}CO_2$ [usually around 28 mm Hg] should not be confused with PetCO$_2$, the partial pressure of end-tidal carbon dioxide [usually between 35 and 40 mm Hg]). This equation indicates that dead space must be large when $PaCO_2$ is much greater than $P\bar{E}CO_2$. The greater the volume of dead space is, the more the carbon dioxide in the exhaled breath ($P\bar{E}CO_2$) will be diluted, or the larger the tidal volume required for a given gradient of arterial-to-mixed exhaled carbon dioxide, the greater the dead space, or the larger the ratio of tidal volume to a given $PaCO_2$, the greater the dead space for a given gradient.

ACCIDENTAL, REAL, OR POTENTIAL DEAD SPACE

In respiratory therapy or anesthesia, when ventilating systems are used that force the patient to inhale premixed gases, the patient could also inhale some exhaled gas containing carbon dioxide. Either by interposing a carbon dioxide absorber and scrubbing the exhaled gas of carbon dioxide (true for anesthesia circle systems) or by arranging for the rapid delivery of fresh gas for every breath (true for most ventilators used in respiratory therapy), rebreathing of carbon dioxide is prevented. It can occur, however, when valves malfunction, when the carbon dioxide absorber in rebreathing systems is exhausted, or when dead space is disproportionately large relative to tidal volume. Rebreathing also can plague the user of systems that rely on high flow rates of fresh gas; these systems (*e.g.*, Mapleson D and Bain) include no carbon dioxide absorber and often have no valves other than a pressure relief valve (pop-off valve.)

INCOMPETENT VALVES

Incompetent valves in anesthesia circle systems can add a significant volume of dead space beyond that of the Y piece if a one-way valve becomes incompetent (Figure 3.1). To demonstrate the effect of an incompetent one-way valve in a circle system anesthesia machine on the capnogram, we infused 250 ml/min of carbon dioxide into an artificial lung with a fan incorporated into the lung to mix gases. We then inserted an endotracheal tube into the "trachea" of the artificial lung, selected a fresh gas flow at a rate of 3 L/min, and ventilated the lung. Then, we rendered the valves incompetent either by inserting a needle between the valve and its seat or by removing the valve entirely.

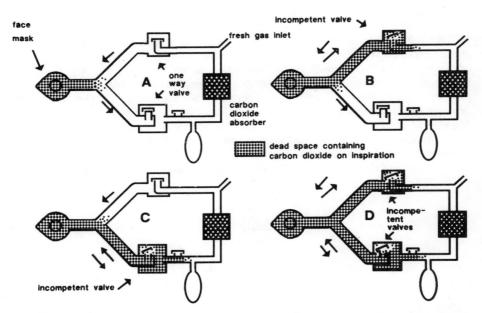

FIGURE 3.1 *Diagram of a circle system. In **A** the circle system is diagrammed with intact valves. The dead space (stippled) is limited to the mask and "Y" piece. In **B** the inspiratory valve is incompetent. The gas deposited in the inspiratory limb during expiration will enlarge the dead space. In **C** the expiratory valve is incompetent and in **D** both valves are. The extent of the added dead space depends on tidal volume, fresh gas flow, and pattern of ventilation (see also Figure 3.5).*

Even a minor incompetence produced by inserting a 25-gauge needle between the valve and its seat was noticeable on the capnogram. Typically, with a leak of either inspiratory (Figure 3.2) or expiratory valve (Figure 3.3), expiratory carbon dioxide values increased. With leaks of only the expiratory valve, values for inspiratory carbon dioxide concentration increased consistently unless the rate of fresh gas flow was extraordinarily high. When the expiratory valve disk was removed, the capnogram became grossly distorted (Figure 3.4).

Rate of fresh gas flow will have an impact on the amount of rebreathing with an incompetent valve if the patient depends on mechanical ventilation during anesthesia with a circle system. The higher the rate of fresh gas flow and the larger the tidal volume, the greater the volume of fresh gas that will be pushed into the lungs,[2] and, therefore, the more diluted the carbon dioxide that is rebreathed. Large effective minute ventilation will also remove more

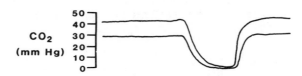

FIGURE 3.2   *Effect on the capnogram of removing the inspiratory valve from an anesthesia circle system. Capnograms (sidestream analyzer) from two identical breaths are superimposed, the lower tracing taken with all valves intact, the upper with the inspiratory valve removed. The lowest inspiratory values are identical, but the expiratory values show rebreathing. Observe that the downslope of the capnogram (inspiration) is slanted, often the first indication of an incompetent inspiratory valve. The reason for the prolonged downslope is readily appreciated when we picture the small amount of carbon dioxide that expiration deposits in the inspiratory limb and that is detected with the next inspiration. Soon, however, all "old" gas is displaced by fresh gas and the capnogram shows zero carbon dioxide late during inspiration.*

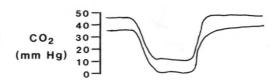

FIGURE 3.3   *Effect on the capnogram of a leaky expiratory valve in an anesthesia circle system. Capnograms (sidestream analyzer) from two identical breaths are superimposed, the lower tracing taken with all valves intact, the upper with a bent 19-gauge needle between the seat of the expiratory valve and the valve disk. This caused the inspiratory carbon dioxide (higher curve) to rise markedly; expiratory carbon dioxide values also increased.*

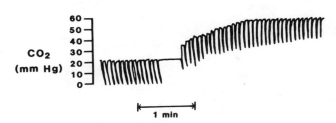

FIGURE 3.4   *Effect on the capnogram of removing the expiratory valve from an anesthesia circle system. Once the expiratory valve is removed, inspiratory and expiratory carbon dioxide increase rapidly with mechanical ventilation (fresh gas flow of 3 L/min) of a mechanical lung (Figures 2.2 and 2.3). (In preparation for photocopying the capnogram was retraced by hand.)*

carbon dioxide, which will be registered on the capnogram. With a leaky valve the capnogram will not be influenced by the rate of fresh gas flow if the patient is breathing spontaneously and as long as neither respiratory rate nor tidal volume is affected by the increasing level of arterial carbon dioxide, which is unlikely.

A brief analysis shows how the type of ventilation system (spontaneous vs. mechanical vs. manually controlled), the rate of fresh gas flow, and the size of the tidal volume can influence the concentration of carbon dioxide when valves leak (Figure 3.5). No gas flows through the Y piece when the patient is not breathing or when the ventilator pauses. During spontaneous ventilation (Figure 3.5A) the excess gas in the system must escape at the end of expiration through the pressure relief (pop-off) valve of the anesthesia circle. Thus, only carbon dioxide-containing gas (not fresh gas) will be vented. With mechanical ventilation (Figure 3.5B) the pressure relief valve of the anesthesia circle must be kept closed, in which case excess gas escapes at the end of expiration through a relief valve incorporated in the ventilator. Again, carbon dioxide-containing gas will be vented, but this gas will be diluted with fresh gas because fresh gas flows from its source into the bellows of the ventilator as the exhaled volume fills the bellows. Thus, with high rates of fresh gas flow this arrangement will vent less carbon dioxide and more fresh gas than would be true with equal gas flow and tidal volume during spontaneous ventilation. With manually controlled ventilation (Figure 3.5C) the pressure relief valve of the anesthesia circle must be kept partly open because the relief valve is the only way that excess gas can escape. Because the highest pressures in these conditions are generated during inspiration, excess gas is vented at that time. This gas will contain not only exhaled carbon dioxide from the expiratory limb of the breathing circle, but also the fresh gas that refills the breathing bag during expiration. Everything else being equal, more carbon dioxide will be rebreathed when the expiratory valve leaks during manual or mechanical ventilation than during spontaneous breathing.

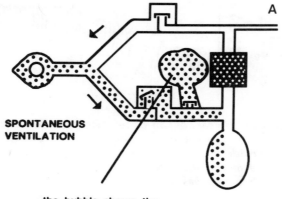

A

**SPONTANEOUS
VENTILATION**

**the bubble shows the
composition of
spilled gas**

THE MORE CARBON DIOXIDE IN THE BUBBLE THE LESS REBREATHING OF CARBON DIOXIDE IN CASE OF VALVE FAILURE

	FRESH GAS
	CARBON DIOXIDE IN EXPIRED GAS

B

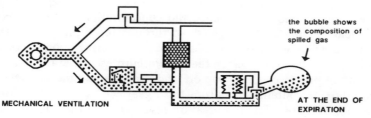

MECHANICAL VENTILATION

the bubble shows
the composition of
spilled gas

**AT THE END OF
EXPIRATION**

at the end of expiration carbon dioxide containing
and fresh gas was spilled through the pressure
relief valve of the ventilator. Therefore more
carbon dioxide was available for reinhalation
than was true for the example with spontaneous
ventilation where only carbon dioxide containing
gas was spilled

C

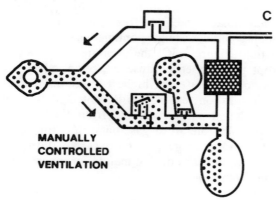

**MANUALLY
CONTROLLED
VENTILATION**

FIGURE 3.5   *Effect on the capnogram of an anesthesia circle system with bag or ventilator and an incompetent expiratory valve. The type of ventilation—spontaneous (A) versus mechanical (B) versus manual (C)—affects the impact of rebreathing when the expiratory valve is incompetent and enables rebreathing. If fresh gas flow rates, volumes of anesthesia machine and ventilator (bag = ventilator bellows), tidal volumes, and physiologic parameters (compliance, resistance, carbon dioxide production, functional residual capacity, and dead space) were all equal with the different systems, the same amount of excess gas would escape from each during one respiratory cycle. With an incompetent expiratory valve more carbon dioxide would be vented (and therefore less would be rebreathed) with spontaneous ventilation than with either mechanical or manually controlled ventilation. The figure does not attempt to quantitate the amount of rebreathing but simply to convey the effect of a leaky expiratory valve on the volume of carbon dioxide spilled.*

NONREBREATHING SYSTEMS

Like most ventilators used in respiratory therapy, the Siemens ventilator used by itself or with the Siemens anesthesia machine has no mechanism for carbon dioxide absorption and therefore no rebreathing occurs. Fresh carbon dioxide-free compressed medical gas flows only during inspiration, and enough fresh gas is delivered with every breath to account for tidal volume. All exhaled gas is vented to the outside. Rebreathing is impossible in these ventilators as long as all valves are competent and as long as the system is correctly assembled. Because rebreathing is theoretically impossible with these systems, capnograms reflect only changes in exhaled gas, inhaled gas containing no carbon dioxide and therefore not needing to be measured. The Siemens capnograph uses the carbon dioxide-free inspiratory phase to recalibrate. (See Part III.)

Semi-open Systems without Valves

A prominent example of nonrebreathing systems is the so-called Bain system, in which fresh gas enters close to the patient's mouth and exhaled gas is breathed into the tube connected to the breathing bag or ventilator. The difficulty with such a system lies in the variability of equipment dead space. It is potentially as great as the breathing tube and the rebreathing bag or ventilator bellows. Only the inflow of fresh gas prevents this potential dead space from becoming a real, external (equipment) dead space. The rate of fresh gas flow can be viewed as being inversely proportional (within limits) to the system dead space: with high fresh gas flow, dead space is small; and with low fresh gas flow, dead space is large (Figure 3.6).

When only small volumes of fresh gas enter the Bain system, the patient is forced to re-inhale large volumes of exhaled gas (Figure 3.6). Fresh gas is continuously blown into the system close to the airway of the patient. The

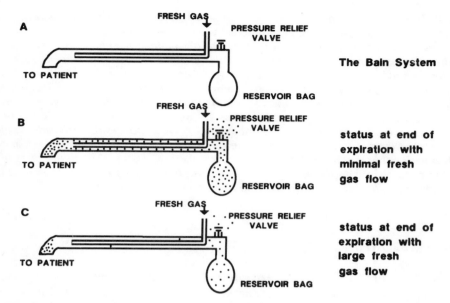

FIGURE 3.6   *The Bain system. The Bain system invites rebreathing with low rates of fresh gas flow. The distribution of carbon dioxide (stippling) at the end of expiration is shown for small (B) and large (C) fresh gas flows.*

exhaled gas fills the external tube and eventually the breathing, or reservoir, bag. A pressure relief valve vents excess gas. At the end of expiration some carbon dioxide is diluted by fresh gas, which continues to flow during expiration and is directed toward the reservoir bag as the patient's lungs are emptying. The next inspiration takes up the fresh gas; if there is not enough to account for inhaled tidal volume, the deficit will be drawn from gas left in the expiratory tube and points beyond. When the fresh gas flow is low (*e.g.*, 2L/min, in an adult), the patient inhales much previously exhaled, carbon dioxide-laden gas. External (equipment or anatomic) dead space will have been considerably enlarged.

At the end of exhalation, with a high rate of fresh gas flow (*e.g.*, 25 L/min for an adult) (Figure 3.6C), not only is much of the exhaled gas washed away, but also the patient receives enough fresh gas throughout the inspiration to prevent rebreathing completely. The patient's dead space will be normal. Many clinicians use values intermediate to the extremes shown here and accept some rebreathing. These observations pertain also to the so-called Mapleson D system, of which the Bain with its coaxial arrangement (fresh gas running through a tube in the center of the breathing conduit) is but a special example.

The complexity of the distribution of carbon dioxide in the Bain system has been analyzed with the help of a computer. Beneken et al.[3] studied the effects on carbon dioxide concentration of volume of the system, compliance of the patient's lungs (for a given pressure during inspiration the tidal volume will be smaller with low compliance and expiration will be faster), carbon dioxide production, setting of the pressure relief valve, tidal volume, respiratory rate, and, most importantly, the rate at which fresh gas flows into the system. All these variables can influence the level of carbon dioxide at the site where it is usually sampled, namely, close to the patient's mouth, and, thus, also influence the shape of the capnogram. If we wish to understand why more or less carbon dioxide returns under different conditions, we can obtain capnograms anywhere in the Bain system. The capnograms from the exhalation tube exhibit shapes that differ strikingly (Figure 3.7).

The coaxial system generates additional problems because of the site where

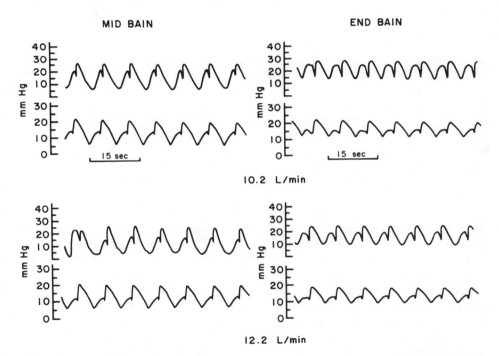

FIGURE 3.7 *Capnograms from the Bain system. The capnogram assumes different shapes depending on where exhaled gas is sampled, the rate of fresh gas flow, the ventilator settings, the volumes of the system, the patient's pulmonary parameters, and the level of carbon dioxide production. Here, experimentally computer-generated capnograms (mechanical lung) reflect gas sampled in the midsection (left) and at the end (right) of the expiratory tube. Fresh gas flow was 10.2 L/min (top four capnograms) and 12.2 L/min (lower four capnograms). The tracings are presented in pairs; the top tracing was obtained experimentally with a mechanical lung (Figure 2.3), and the bottom tracing was generated by a computer. (Reproduced with permission from Beneken JEW, Gravenstein N, Gravenstein JS, et al: Capnography and the Bain circuit I: A computer model. J Clin Monit 1:108, 1985.)*

fresh gas flows into the system. The fresh gas may wash over the sampling site and thus dilute the sample.[4,5] When sidestream analyzers are used for small patients, the sampling flow adds to the difficulty in obtaining representative capnograms of end-tidal carbon dioxide concentrations.[6]

ENVIRONMENTAL CONSIDERATIONS

Recently, we noted the birth of the 5 billionth human being on earth. If every one of us were to rest and produce only 200 ml/min of carbon dioxide, the daily carbon dioxide production would amount to 1,000,000,000 L/min, or 60 billion L/h, or over 525 trillion L/yr. One shudders to think by how much this figure would have to be multiplied if all the carbon dioxide produced by other mammals and animals were to be included in the estimate. Fortunately, carbon dioxide is consumed by green plants. Over the eons, carbon dioxide in the atmosphere has varied widely; just within the past 160,000 years, the level of carbon dioxide has ranged from 0.0178 volume percent, which occurred about 46,000 years ago, to a high of 0.03 volume percent, which is the level at the present time,[7] combustion and chemical reactions from human industry likely contributing prodigious amounts. Indeed, these unnaturally large sources of carbon dioxide have been blamed for an increase in atmospheric levels of carbon dioxide over the years; by 2000 AD, the level of carbon dioxide in the atmosphere is estimated to be 18% higher than that in 1900 AD.

Carbon dioxide that is not taken up by plants is distributed in the enormous mantle of air that surrounds the earth; also, much carbon dioxide is dissolved in the oceans, rivers, and lakes. When we are forced to live in a closed space cut off from such natural outlets for carbon dioxide, because of our incessant production of carbon dioxide, it will accumulate in the confined space, for example, as occurs in submarines and space capsules. Because scrubbing such systems of all carbon dioxide taxes the energy resources and weight limitations of self-contained systems, submarine crews and astronauts must tolerate a slightly elevated level of carbon dioxide in the air they breathe. Levels between 0.7 and 1.2 volume percent carbon dioxide in the inspired gas are well tolerated; with exercise, the levels may rise to about 2%. When this level reaches 3%, breathing masks are worn. In submarines and space ships, the carbon dioxide levels are carefully monitored. Indeed, the introduction into clinical medicine of some monitoring techniques, for example, mass spectrometry, has greatly benefited from the developments in submarine and space craft applications.

Even when closed, most windows and doors of rooms in homes and hospitals allow for the circulation of air. However, when many people assemble in rooms with windows and doors closed, such as can happen in lecture rooms, the carbon dioxide levels may rise markedly, perhaps to 0.5% or more, depending on circumstances. That carbon dioxide accumulates in closed spaces needs to be taken into account when calibrating capnometers that are manufactured on the assumption that ambient gas is always practically free of carbon dioxide.

REFERENCES

1. West JB: Ventilation-Blood Flow and Gas Exchange, ed 2. Oxford, Blackwell, 1970
2. Gravenstein N, Banner MJ, McLaughlin G: Tidal volume changes due to the interaction of anesthesia machine and anesthesia ventilator. J Clin Monit 3:187–190, 1987
3. Beneken JEW, Gravenstein N, Gravenstein JS, et al: Capnography and the Bain circuit. I. A computer model. J Clin Monit 1:103–113, 1985
4. Kaplan RF, Paulus DA: Error in sampling of exhaled gases. Anesth Analg 62:955–956, 1983
5. Gravenstein N, Lampotang S, Beneken JEW: Factors influencing capnography in the Bain circuit. J Clin Monit 1:6–10, 1985
6. Schieber RA, Namnoum A, Sugden A, et al: Accuracy of expiratory carbon dioxide measurements using the coaxial and circle breathing circuits in small subjects. J Clin Monit 1:149–155, 1985
7. Barnola JM, Raynaud D, Korotkevich YS, et al: Vostok ice core provides 160,000-year record of atmospheric CO_2. Nature 329:408–414, 1987

Chapter 4

Clinical Indications

Capnography has been used in anesthesia and respiratory therapy for many years and, in some countries (for instance The Netherlands), has become a requisite in routine anesthesia. Recently, American clinicians have been reexamining the role of capnography, and now this monitoring method is rapidly gaining in use. Even the American Society of Anesthesiologists (ASA) in 1986 formally encouraged the use of capnography in clinical anesthesia.[1] Capnography enhances safety and facilitates mechanical ventilation and diagnosis in the operating room and intensive care unit.

SAFETY

In recent years some of the most devastating disasters in anesthesia have been linked to problems with ventilation. Capnography, therefore, has received much attention because carbon dioxide detected in a patient's exhaled gas gives evidence of ventilation. There may be too much carbon dioxide, too little, or just the right amount, but at least we know respiration has not stopped if a capnogram is being traced. Further, because the method is inexpensive and relatively easy to institute, capnography can be used as a basic safety monitor.

Intubation of Trachea vs. Esophagus

Statistics indicate that esophageal (instead of tracheal) intubation has caused many disasters.[2] Experienced clinicians are not astonished. Ascertaining whether the endotracheal tube has been properly inserted into the trachea or improperly into the esophagus is often vexingly difficult. During the intubation itself, in some cases it may be difficult or impossible to observe the tip of the endotracheal tube going into the larynx, in which case we auscultate the chest while we compress the reservoir bag. However, in obese patients breath sounds are often difficult to hear; thus, we watch for condensation to form in the endotracheal tube during exhalation; unfortunately, gas issuing from the esophagus and stomach might also generate condensation. A smart push on the patient's chest may cause a tangible puff of gas to come out of the endotracheal tube, a puff that is sometimes insignificant and difficult to sense. Over the trachea just below the cricoid cartilage, we feel for the cuff of the endotracheal tube by inflating and deflating the cuff repeatedly. Feeling a bulge through the tracheal ring when the cuff is inflated reassures us that the tube is not inserted too far, but we can be fooled. In a slender patient a bulging cuff that we think is extending the trachea may actually lie in the esophagus. We listen over the stomach for the sound of bubbling gas while we compress the reservoir bag. Sometimes the gas either makes little noise or does not even go into the stomach but instead flows retrograde out of the esophagus and from there to the trachea.

Is there a way to know whether the tube is really in the trachea? Yes—through capnography. The capnogram cannot show whether the tube has been pushed too far down the trachea and has entered a mainstem bronchus or has not been pushed far enough and teeters precariously at the larynx, ready to slip out. Repeated upstrokes in the capnogram do show ventilation of the alveoli, which means there is an avenue for oxygenation. Theoretically, it is possible to sample carbon dioxide-containing gas from the stomach. A gas bubble in the stomach will be made up of swallowed gas, which eventually equilibrates with blood gases. During mechanical ventilation, the stomach can be inflated with either fresh gas or gas that contains carbon dioxide. But even in the most unfavorable conditions, ventilation of the stomach cannot yield a capnogram comparable to that after tracheal intubation. In an animal experiment, carbon dioxide-containing gas was blown into the stomach and the stomach was then ventilated through a long tube inserted into the stomach itself. The end-tidal carbon dioxide concentration in the resulting capnogram declined quickly to an insignificant level (Figure 4.1). A normal capnogram inscribed after successful intubation is one of the sweetest sights for the anesthetist.

Apnea

When a patient suffers a respiratory arrest, a capnograph sounds an alarm when the next wave of carbon dioxide fails to arrive. Here we must distinguish between the workings of sidestream analyzers and mainstream analyzers. When respiration is arrested, a sidestream analyzer soon detects no carbon dioxide; the capnogram will return to zero because the sidestream analyzer aspirates gas continuously. Whatever carbon dioxide had been left in the sampling connector of the sidestream analyzer will eventually be aspirated by the analyzer and replaced with fresh gas. With the mainstream analyzer, whether the arrest occurred during inspiration (when fresh gas is under the sensor and the capnogram thus continues to show no carbon dioxide) or during expiration (the carbon dioxide registered during expiration remains stationary because no fresh gas displaces it), the carbon dioxide diffuses and the capnogram dwindles. Both sidestream and mainstream capnographs, however, will sound an alarm when

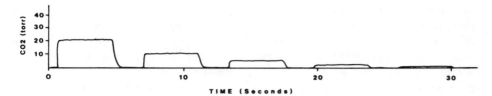

TIME (Seconds)

FIGURE 4.1   *Capnogram obtained from an anesthetized dog after esophageal intubation. Observe the declining end-tidal values. (Courtesy of Drs. ML Good and JH Modell, University of Florida.)*

another breath fails to arrive. The time from apnea to alarm (often adjustable, but usually less than 15 sec) varies with the model of capnograph.

Capnographic monitoring for apnea is especially beneficial for patients in the postanesthesia care unit. These patients are predisposed to respiratory failure because modern anesthetic techniques still depend on respiratory depressants: potent narcotics and muscle relaxants. In particular jeopardy are patients with preexisting pulmonary disease or obesity who undergo anesthesia, especially narcotic-relaxant anesthesia for upper abdominal and thoracic operations.

Capnographs easily monitor apnea when a patient's trachea is intubated. Using capnography to monitor an unintubated, spontaneously breathing patient is more difficult. Simply positioning the sampling tube near the nares or the mouth has certain limitations. With sidestream analyzers gases can be sampled from a patient's nose (for instance by attaching the collecting capillary to the nasal prongs normally used to administer oxygen) or from the nasopharynx by inserting an aspirating tube through a nostril; with this technique, however, secretions frequently obstruct the tube. There have been some recent improvements, however.[3,4] One simple solution is to use a nasal cannula cut to fit into the sampling catheter lumen. Another solution is placement of a nasal airway with the sampling catheter positioned concentrically and sutured in place.[5] All these manipulations require that the end of the sampling catheter be placed back from the end of the nasal cannula or from the pharyngeal opening.

Sampling from a disposable oxygen mask has also been suggested.[6] A 14-gauge, 1.25-inch catheter is inserted through a side port at a point close to the nose. The catheter is secured to the mask with adhesive tape and connected to the sampling line of the mass spectrometer. This has the advantage of not being susceptible to the accumulation of secretions.

In using any of these alternatives, sample flow rate is an important variable to consider. With the face-mask alternative, mainstream or sidestream sampling is compatible with 15- to 22-mm adaptors.

Many ophthalmologic procedures are performed with local anesthesia. Many of these patients are elderly people undergoing a cataract operation, which necessitates that a drape cover the entire face, except for the eye being operated on. We use nasal prongs to administer oxygen (2 to 4 L/min) and we tape the sampling capillary to the chin so that the end lies close to the lower lip (Figure 4.2). With this arrangement the mass spectrometer detected a higher concentration of expired than inspired oxygen (Figure 4.3). During expiration supplemental oxygen being delivered to the patient was blown into the area where gas was sampled. During inspiration there were two sources of carbon dioxide. First, a small amount remained around the patient's mouth where gas was sampled. Second, because high rates of flow through nasal cannula can irritate nasal mucosa, nasal oxygen was delivered at a flow rate of 2 L/min, far less than minute ventilation; therefore, inspired air was likely to have contained gas from around the mouth and hence some carbon dioxide. Carbon dioxide under the drapes can be lowered by blowing several liters of air or oxygen under the drapes or by using a vacuum tube to remove gas, this gas then being replaced by room air as it diffuses into the space.

MONITORING ADEQUACY OF MECHANICAL VENTILATION

In all patients who depend on mechanical ventilation tidal volume and respiratory rate must be adjusted to attain a particular level of end-tidal carbon

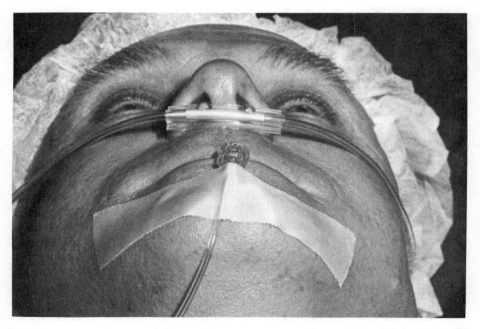

FIGURE 4.2   *Capnographic sampling during spontaneous breathing. A sampling catheter of a sidestream analyzer can be attached to a patient's chin (or upper lip) when, for instance, the face will be covered by drapes during an opthalmologic operation. Nasal prongs have been inserted to administer oxygen.*

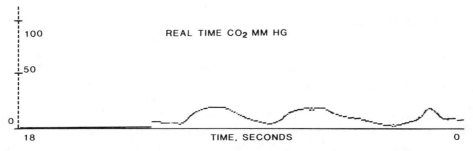

PATIENT ID:

STATION # 5 DATA @ 08:46   07/07/87   08:47
STNS MON   3   5   13 14   REPT SCAN:
             CO₂   O₂   N₂   N₂O   HAL   ENF   ISO
INSP MM   2.92   163.2   541.8   .0   .00   .00   .00
EXP MM   18.39   274.5   413.5   .0   .00   .00   .00
RESP   @   PRINTING
BLOOD   PH   @
RESP RATE: 15.3   I : E : 1: .77   EXP. TIME: 1.7

FIGURE 4.3 *Capnogram from patient breathing spontaneously under drapes. The patient was undergoing a cataract operation with local anesthesia. Oxygen was administered by nasal prongs and expired and inspired gases were monitored (Figure 4.2). Observe that inspired oxygen is lower than expired oxygen.*

dioxide tension. When patients require mechanical ventilation, the initial minute ventilation is usually based on a formula (for instance 10 to 12 ml/kg with a respiratory rate of 10 breaths/min), or a nomogram is used. However, neither formula nor nomogram can take into account the many factors that may modify respiratory requirements. It is therefore helpful to monitor end-tidal carbon dioxide. Adherence to formula and nomogram usually brings end-tidal values close to the expected, and only small adjustments are needed to attain the desired value. If large adjustments are called for, an explanation for the discrepancy is in order. Is the patient producing carbon dioxide at an abnormal rate? Is alveolar dead space increased? Is the capnograph functioning properly? Whenever there are questions about the possibility of a shunt, whether anatomic (right-to-left shunt secondary to cardiac lesions or injury) or functional ($\dot{V}/\dot{Q}$ abnormalities based on anesthetic drugs, position, surgical interference with the lung, or pulmonary disease), capnography must be supplemented by arterial blood gas analysis, including both oxygen and carbon dioxide. (See Part II for details.)

In a few instances the demands for adjusting minute ventilation are very specific. During neurosurgical procedures, particularly with space-occupying lesions, proper anesthetic care often includes lowering the arterial carbon dioxide tension in order to make use of the interaction between carbon dioxide and brain blood flow to control intracranial volume and pressure. Also, in patients undergoing cardiopulmonary bypass, accidental hyperventilation before perfusion and increased central venous pressure caused by fluctuating arterial carbon dioxide tension immediately after perfusion is begun may result in neurologic deficit.[7] In modern anesthesia such procedures are no longer performed without measuring carbon dioxide, either in arterial blood or end-tidal gas. Capnography offers by far the most convenient and continuous method to monitor carbon dioxide levels. Yet it may be necessary to compare end-tidal levels against arterial levels in order to rule out abnormal arterial-to-alveolar carbon dioxide gradients.

MALIGNANT HYPERTHERMIA

Malignant hyperthermia syndrome requires oxygen consumption and carbon dioxide production to increase before temperature can rise. Therefore, monitoring carbon dioxide tension or concentration in the expired gas recommends itself as a sensitive variable in the diagnosis of malignant hyperthermia. How striking the changes in end-tidal carbon dioxide concentration can be has been illustrated in a number of case reports, *e.g.*, a 4-year-old boy reported by Dunn et al.[8] The little patient was anesthetized uneventfully with halothane, nitrous oxide, and oxygen after intubation with the help of succinylcholine. After 2 hours of anesthesia the patient began to hyperventilate and end-tidal carbon dioxide levels increased within 10 minutes from 30 mm Hg to 90 mm Hg. During the previous hour temperature had only increased from 35.2°C to 37°C. Thus, unexpected increases in end-tidal carbon dioxide tension must quickly raise the suspicion of malignant hyperthermia, a condition that requires early diagnosis and vigorous treatment, which in the case noted here included dantrolene and supportive measures.

COMA

In patients with head trauma, the clinician must expect respiratory depression and elevated arterial carbon dioxide blood tensions. Indeed, arterial carbon dioxide tensions measured early after head trauma correlated strongly: the more serious the trauma, as judged by the Glasgow coma scale, the greater the elevation of arterial carbon dioxide.[9] Monitoring ventilation and end-tidal or arterial carbon dioxide is essential in the comatose patient, whether the coma is caused by trauma or other reasons.

REFERENCES

1. Eichhorn JH: ASA adopts basic monitoring standards. Anesthesia Patient Safety Foundation Newsletter 2:1–3, March 1987
2. Cheney FW: What is anesthesia? Potential risks, causes of incidents, in Gravenstein JS, Holzer JF (eds): Safety and Cost Containment in Anesthesia. Boston, Butterworths, 1988, pp 11–20

3. Ibarra E, Lees DE: Mass spectrometer monitoring of patients with regional anesthesia. Anesthesiology 63:572–573, 1985
4. Goldman JM: A simple, easy, and inexpensive method for monitoring $ETCO_2$ through nasal cannulae. Anesthesiology 67:606, 1987
5. Norman EA, Zeig NJ, Ahmad I: Better designs for mass spectrometer monitoring of the awake patient. Anesthesiology 64:664, 1986
6. Huntington CT, King HK: A simpler design for mass spectrometer monitoring of the awake patient. Anesthesiology 65:565–566, 1986
7. Nevin M, Adams S, Colchester ACF, et al: Evidence for involvement of hypocapnia and hypoperfusion in aetiology of neurological deficit after cardiopulmonary bypass. Lancet 2:1493–1495, 1987
8. Dunn CM, Maltry DE, Eggers GWN Jr: Value of mass spectrometry in early diagnosis of malignant hyperthermia. Anesthesiology 68:333, 1985
9. Pfenninger E, Ahnefeld FW, Kilian J, et al: Das Verhalten der Blutgase bei Schädel-Hirn-traumatisierten Patienten am Unfallort und bei der Klinikaufnahme. Anaesthesist 36:570–576, 1987

PART II

Physiologic Perspectives on Carbon Dioxide

Chapter 5

Production of Carbon Dioxide

Capnometry, by estimating the level of partial pressure, or tension, of carbon dioxide in arterial blood, often expressed as $PaCO_2$, guides clinicians in assessing the adequacy of ventilation and alerts us to changes in circulation and metabolism. Carbon dioxide also influences cerebral blood flow; as $PaCO_2$ rises, cerebral blood flow increases because arteries dilate, and as $PaCO_2$ decreases, the arteries constrict. In neurosurgical anesthesia we use this interaction to reduce brain volume. However, excessive hypocapnia itself may have deleterious effects on the brain,[1] presumably because the supply of nutrients and oxygen becomes less than the demand. Elevated levels of arterial carbon dioxide also affect the peripheral circulation by causing vasodilation of beds not constricted by sympathetic influences while stimulating the sympathetic nervous system and, thus, causing constriction of vascular beds that are innervated.

The clinically important factors that affect carbon dioxide are metabolism, which generates carbon dioxide; blood and circulation, which transport carbon dioxide; and, finally, ventilation, which eliminates carbon dioxide from the body. Factors that affect the levels of carbon dioxide in the alveoli are metabolic rate, alveolar ventilation, and the ventilation-to-perfusion ratio of the lungs. Factors that affect alveolar carbon dioxide indirectly include the respiratory quotient (RQ), diffusion of gas and its transport in blood, and acid–base balance.

INFLUENCES ON CARBON DIOXIDE PRODUCTION

Aerobic metabolism, over many intermediate steps, generates carbon dioxide and water (Figure 5.1). The process starts with the uptake of glucose and oxygen by the cell and ends with the generation of energy and the elimination of carbon dioxide. A number of conditions and diseases can influence the consumption of oxygen, which has commensurate effects on the metabolism of substrate and the production of carbon dioxide.

53

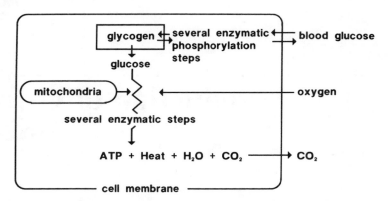

FIGURE 5.1   *Cellular generation of carbon dioxide. This simplified scheme shows that oxygen and substrate enter the cell, that the mitochondria play a pivotal role in generating energy and heat from the substrate, and that carbon dioxide and water leave the cell.*

Mitochondrial Diseases

Increased Production of Carbon Dioxide

The mitochondria, the factory that controls the fires that burn about 80% of the oxygen supply, produce most endogenous carbon dioxide. The best known mitochondrial defect is hyperthyroidism, which markedly accelerates mitochondrial oxygen consumption of most cells except for erythrocytes and cells in the brain, spleen, and testis; carbon dioxide production and energy generation keep pace with the increased oxygen consumption. Two other, much rarer mitochondrial disorders not involving thyroid hormones but associated with accelerated oxygen consumption and carbon dioxide production are Luft's disease, which affects calcium transport in muscle,[2] and Vera's disease,[3] associated with pathologic muscle contraction resistant to neuromuscular blocking drugs.

When oxygen consumption and carbon dioxide production are either normal or increased but energy production is lower than normal, we speak of uncoupling; oxidation of substrate proceeds, but the generation of high-energy adenosine triphosphate (ATP) lags behind. A typical example is severe salicylate poisoning: oxygen consumption may be brisk, not only because of coexisting hyperpyrexia, but also because of mitochrondrial effects, but oxidation is dissociated, uncoupled, from phosphorylation.[4] Finally, the Kearns-Sayre syndrome must be mentioned (the so-called ragged fiber disease because of the microscopic appearance in muscle mitochondria), a myopathy associated with a marked increase of oxygen consumption and often a concomitant lactic acidosis, as well as defects in the eyes and heart.[5]

Another latent muscle disease, *i.e.,* malignant hyperthermia or malignant familial hyperpyrexia, kills its victims with a raging fever accompanied by a drastic acceleration of oxygen consumption and carbon dioxide production. Anesthesiologists in particular are greatly concerned with this genetic disease, which can be unleashed by certain anesthetic agents. In patients genetically at risk the administration of succinylcholine and a halogenated anesthetic such as halothane at the same time can trigger the syndrome. These patients may become stiff with muscle rigidity, often most pronounced or first noticed in the masseters, and, paradoxically, often elicited by the depolarizing neuromuscular blocking drug succinylcholine. Tachycardia, arrhythmia, and severe metabolic acidosis follow. The incidence of this syndrome, terrifying in its sudden and drastic nature, is fortunately low, accounting for about 1 in 15,000 patients who undergo anesthesia. Malignant hyperpyrexia can be treated or, when anticipated because of a telling family or personal history, prevented with dantrolene, which retards the release of calcium from the sarcoplasmic reticulum and, thus, reduces muscle contraction.

A substantial, otherwise unexplained increase in end-tidal carbon dioxide during general anesthesia has, at times, been the first indication that malignant hyperpyrexia was imminent.[6] Capnography has therefore been advocated in the routine monitoring of patients at risk for hyperpyrexia.

Decreased Production of Carbon Dioxide

Hypothyroidism, the first metabolic problem to come to mind that decreases carbon dioxide production, is generally well known. It is essentially an inverse mirror of hyperthyroidism. Patients with muscular dystrophies or with Reye's syndrome (encephalopathy and liver failure)[7] appear to have mitochondrial abnormalities associated with decreases in oxygen consumption and carbon dioxide production.

Cyanide intoxication deserves discussion among anesthesiologists, intensivists, and internists. Cyanide inhibits the cytochromes a_1 and a_3 of all but red blood cells. This poisoning is a common effect of ingestion of the cassava root (Manihot esculenta *Crantz)* in Africa and often associated with tropical ataxic neuropathy. Rarer is cyanide poisoning from apricot pits and chokecherries and, fortunately, equally rare, from a criminal act.

The clinical administration of sodium nitroprusside may inadvertently lead to cyanide intoxication; typical signs consist of hyperventilation (if the patient is not paralyzed and mechanically ventilated), nausea, dizziness, drowsiness, and, eventually, convulsions. In anesthetized patients these symptoms are obscured, and the diagnosis is vexing. Blood pressure values are difficult to interpret because sodium nitroprusside is used in these patients specifically to control high arterial pressure or to induce hypotension. One clue to cyanide intoxication is metabolic acidosis; as the poisoned mitochondrial machinery slows, oxygen consumption and carbon dioxide production decrease. The interference in aerobic metabolism leads inevitably to metabolic acidosis. Because less oxygen is consumed, mixed venous oxygen tension will increase until cardiac output decreases dramatically. Therefore, monitoring cardiac output and oxygen content or partial pressure of oxygen in pulmonary arterial blood (which reflects mixed venous blood) can prove helpful. The diagnosis is verified by measuring blood thiocyanate, a metabolite of nitroprusside. Thiocyanate blood levels less than 10 mg/dl are usually well tolerated. For an immediate effect, as required for induced hypotension during anesthesia, the total dose of nitroprusside administered over 3 hours is best kept lower than 1 mg/kg. For the average adult weighing 70 kg, the infusion rate should be about 300 μg/min. For more protracted treatment with sodium nitroprusside, lower rates of infusion are used, *i.e.,* 200 μg/kg/h or about 200 μg/min.[8]

METABOLIC INFLUENCES

Respiratory Quotient

The production of carbon dioxide parallels the consumption of oxygen, glucose, and other substrate. With no substrate, there is no carbon dioxide production. This chain reaction is of great interest to the clinician not only because of the energy required to run the physiologic machinery, but also because the cycle varies with the substrate. For instance, when glucose alone is metabolized, for every molecule of oxygen consumed, one molecule of carbon dioxide results. The ratio of carbon dioxide production to oxygen consumption, or carbon dioxide production divided by oxygen consumption, is called the respiratory quotient (RQ) (Table 5.1). The RQ is actually an average value for the RQs of all organs. The brain, which depends heavily on glucose, can have a different RQ from the liver, which metabolizes proteins or fat. Based on blood flow to each organ and its oxygen extraction per milliliter of blood, the RQ of one organ may contribute more or less than that of another organ to the average RQ.

The RQ also varies with diet and time of day. After a meal when carbohydrates are metabolized, the RQ approaches 1.0. Hours after a meal or during fasting, when carbohydrates are exhausted, RQ falls to a little over 0.7. The glycogen stores in liver and muscle normally amount to only a few hundred grams. When these preferred carbohydrate stores for metabolism are exhausted, the body begins to consume fat and proteins, some of which are converted to glucose to satisfy the metabolic requirements of the brain. Thus, patients who must undergo protracted fasts, because of disease or preparation for surgical operation, will have low RQs. Another group who have low RQs are diabetic patients whose disease is poorly controlled and whose blood sugar levels, therefore, are high because fats, rather than carbohydrates, are metabolized.

The RQ of an average patient usually hovers around 0.85. Whether it fluctuates slightly has no influence on most clinical decisions and treatment plans. The RQ does become important in certain patients receiving parenteral

Table 5.1 Respiratory Quotients for Oxidation of Different Substrates

Substrate	Chemical Formula	Metabolic End Product	Ratio of Carbon Dioxide to Oxygen	Respiratory Quotient
Glucose	$C_6H_{12}O_6 + 6 O_2$	$6 CO_2 + 6 H_2O$	6/6	1.00
Triolein	$C_{57}H_{104}O_6 + 80 O_2$	$57 CO_2 + 52 H_2O$	57/80	0.71
Alanine	$2C_3H_7O_2N + 6 O_2$	$(NH_2)_2CO + 5 CO_2 + 5 H_2O$	5/6	0.83

Reproduced with permission from Guyton AC: Textbook of Medical Physiology, ed 5. Philadelphia, WB Saunders, 1976, p 972.

nutrition. Most formulas for parenteral (and even enteral) nutrients for critically ill patients contain more carbohydrates than other nutrients and therefore push RQ toward 1.0. To consider the metabolic effects, assume that a critically ill adult is suffering from a pulmonary disease with respiratory insufficiency. Substituting 30% fat for carbohydrate would reduce the RQ and, thus, the minute ventilation necessary to maintain normal $PaCO_2$.[9] Thus, not only tidal volume, respiratory rate, and fraction of oxygen in inspired gas, but also diet can be adjusted to the advantage of patients with respiratory insufficiency.

A further consideration in this contest is that strenuous exercise or formation of lipids can increase the RQ to greater than 1.0. During strenuous exercise and anaerobic metabolism, lactate levels in blood rise and bicarbonate levels fall; intracellular pH falls. After discontinuation of exercise, the elimination of carbon dioxide proceeds more slowly than oxygen is consumed and the RQ rises transiently above 1.0.[10] The RQ can also exceed 1.0 when lipids are formed from glucose because the conversion of glucose, which contains much oxygen (observe the general formula of $C_6H_{12}O_{12}$), into lipids, which do not (observe for example the general formula for triolein, $C_{57}H_{104}O_6$), over many intermediate steps liberates the excess oxygen contained in glucose.

Basal Metabolic Rate

A link between oxygen consumption (and hence carbon dioxide production) and temperature (Figure 5.1) enables oxygen consumption to produce energy, which in turn can be expressed in calories. A calorie (with a lowercase c) is the amount of heat needed to warm 1 g of water from 15°C to 16°C (or 59°F to 61°F). A more recent and preferred convention defines 1 calorie as 4.18 joules. In clinical calorimetry, we reckon with thousands of calories and therefore use the kilocalorie (sometimes also called the kilogramcalorie), usually written as Calorie (with a capital C), which represents 1000 calories. The so-called basal metabolic rate (BMR) expressed in Calories consumed per hour by a resting adult is about 1 Calorie/h/kg of body weight. The BMR is commonly estimated by recording the volume of oxygen consumed under the assumption that more than 95% of metabolic energy is extracted from the oxidation of substrate. Under this assumption 4.6 to 5.06 Calories are generated by every liter of oxygen, depending on whether protein, fat, or carbohydrates were metabolized. A useful average is that about 4.8 Calories are generated with every liter of oxygen consumed or, postulating an RQ of 0.85, with every 850 ml of carbon dioxide produced. Average BMR values for normal adults have been tabulated in a number of nomograms.[11]

Those factors that influence carbon dioxide production also influence average BMR values in the same direction. For instance hypothyroidism, Addison's disease, eunuchoidism, myotonia atrophica, and the nephrotic syndrome would lower the BMR. An increase in BMR occurs with hyperthyroidism, pheochromocytoma, hyperpituitarism, untreated tetanus, and conditions associated with persistent fever such as chronic as well as granulocytic leukemia, tuberculosis, and certain tumors with much mitotic activity.

Several conditions that occur in acutely ill patients in operating rooms and intensive care units also modify the BMR that would normally be expected (Tables 5.2 and 5.3). The calculation of energy requirement invites an interesting calculation of glucose requirement in the resting adult or in an anesthetized patient. Assume that you are anesthetizing an average adult and that he generates carbon dioxide at 200 ml/min; therefore, he will produce carbon dioxide at 12 L/h ($200 \times 60 = 12,000$ ml). Assuming an RQ of 1.0, he will also consume that many liters of oxygen during that time and, metabolizing the equivalent of 5.06 Calories/L of oxygen, he will generate about 61 Calories/h. The metabolism of glucose generates, per gram mole, about 686 Calories. The generation of 61 Calories therefore would call for the metabolism of 0.09 moles of glucose. One mole of glucose (anhydrous) equals 180 g. Every hour our anesthetized man will therefore metabolize 16.2 g of glucose. If it were administered intravenously, this would call for 324 ml/h of dextrose 5% in

Table 5.2 Estimation of Energy Requirements by Body Weight

	Body Weight (kg)						
	50	55	60	65	70	75	80
Basal metabolic rate (Calorie/day)	1316	1411	1509	1602	1699	1784	1872
Oxygen consumed (ml/min)	189	203	217	231	245	257	269
Carbon dioxide produced (ml/min)	161	173	184	196	208	218	229

Formula for the daily energy requirement for weight maintenance: normal basal metabolic rate × modifying factor (see Table 5.3). (Modified with permission from Wilmore DW: Enteral and parenteral nutrition in hospital patients. Sci Am Med 14:2, 1984.)

Table 5.3 Modifying Factor of Some Pathophysiologic Conditions in Calculating the Basal Metabolic Rate

Condition	Modifying Factor
Mild starvation	0.85–1.00
Normal postoperative recovery	1.00–1.05
Peritonitis	1.05–1.25
Cancer	1.10–1.45
Severe infection or multiple trauma	1.30–1.55

The modifying factor must be increased by another 20% to 25% in patients who are active or stressed by therapeutic interventions. The modifying factor will also be influenced by the extent of the disease, infection, or trauma. The data, therefore, are general guides rather than specific values for each patient. (Modified with permission from Wilmore DW: Enteral and parenteral nutrition in hospital patients. Sci Am Med 14:2, 1984.)

water. This is not a therapeutic recommendation because the RQ and many other factors have to be taken into account when intraoperative fluid therapy is prescribed, but this exercise illuminates the order of magnitude of oxygen consumption, carbon dioxide production, and glucose utilization in anesthetized patients.

A question from a different point of view is whether administering glucose intraoperatively would influence carbon dioxide production and the RQ immediately after operation. From data collected in a postanesthesia care unit (Table 5.4),[12] we may conclude that the administration of glucose intraoperatively, on the one hand, increased carbon dioxide production and, on the other, provided the metabolic substrate that (judging from RQ) would otherwise have been taken from protein and lipids. Again, we are reminded that metabolism can influence ventilation, which is critically important in patients with respiratory insufficiency.

Temperature

It is well appreciated that hypothermia substantially decreases oxygen consumption and hence, also, carbon dioxide production. Hibernation is a positive application of this relationship; animals consume much less oxygen and substrate and, of course, generate and use much less energy during their long winter sleep. Conversely, metabolism increases with exercise and fever. It is little appreciated that nothing more than excitement may cause a fever of 38°C in a few individuals. In many, temperature may decrease to less than 36°C during normal sleep; on awakening, metabolism must be elevated to restore normal body temperature. During these transitions—from abnormally low during cool slumber to abnormally high with excitement—oxygen consumption and carbon dioxide production may increase more than the level of core temperature suggests. Once a steady state is reached, the amount of oxygen

Table 5.4 The Effect of Saline vs. Glucose Infusion during Anesthesia on Respiratory Quotient and Carbon Dioxide Production in the Recovery Room

Intraoperative Intravenous Fluids	Metabolism in the Recovery Room	
	Average Respiratory Quotient	*Average Carbon Dioxide Production (ml/min)*
Glucose	0.93	175
Saline	0.77	150

(Modified from Hagerdal M, Caldwell CB, Gross JB: Intraoperative fluid management influences carbon dioxide production and respiratory quotient. Anesthesiology 59:48–50, 1983.)

consumed and carbon dioxide produced during hypothermia or fever can be measured.

As a rule of thumb, at steady state a rise or fall by 1°C will cause a parallel change in oxygen consumption by about 7%. Thus, in a 75-kg adult with a fever of 39°C, oxygen consumption would increase from a normal resting rate of approximately 260 ml/min at 37°C to about 300 ml/min; the same person undergoing hypothermic anesthesia with a core temperature of 30°C might consume only 126 ml/min of oxygen. These figures are calculated averages and depend on many additional circumstances, *e.g.*, anesthesia. At the conclusion of anesthesia, a very unsteady state exists. If a patient's core temperature had decreased during anesthesia by as little as 1°C, normal body temperature may be restored in the recovery room by vigorous shivering and doubling of oxygen consumption.[13] Carbon dioxide production and ventilatory requirements, in lockstep with oxygen consumption, would also double at the same rate.

We can grasp the magnitude of changes in carbon dioxide production, oxygen consumption, and, hence, ventilatory requirements effected by shifts in temperature, but we cannot precisely calculate or predict these changes during anesthesia, operation, or other treatment; too many variables influence metabolism under these stressful conditions.

Shivering

The body temperature of many patients cools during operations in cold operating rooms, and particularly so when body cavities or large wounds are exposed for protracted times. Who has not seen a shivering patient in the recovery room? However, apparently not all shivering can be explained by a decreased temperature. Regardless of the mechanism, during shivering oxygen consumption and carbon dioxide production increase markedly (Table 5.5).[13] Whether suppression of shivering should be attempted with drugs depends on the clinical circumstances.

INFLUENCES OF ANESTHESIA AND MUSCLE RELAXATION

It would seem obvious that anesthesia and muscle relaxation should reduce the metabolic requirements for oxygen, but that is not necessarily the case. In carefully controlled animal experiments the lowest oxygen consumption ($\dot{V}O_2$) occurred during normal sleep ($\dot{V}O_2 = 2.46$ ml $\cdot$ kg^{-1} $\cdot$ min^{-1}).[14] With different agents oxygen consumption actually increased during deep anesthesia (to about $\dot{V}O_2 = 3.45$ ml $\cdot$ kg^{-1} $\cdot$ min^{-1} with mechanical ventilation and to 4.5 ml $\cdot$ kg^{-1} $\cdot$ min^{-1} with spontaneous ventilation). When the animals were alert and resting, oxygen consumption was a little higher still ($\dot{V}O_2 = 5.5$ ml $\cdot$kg^{-1} $\cdot$ min^{-1}).

Table 5.5 The Effect of Medication to Prevent Postoperative Shivering

	Shivering	*Shivering Blocked by Meperidine*
Oxygen consumption (L · min^{-1} · 70 kg^{-1} STPD)	0.93	0.38
Carbon dioxide production (L · min^{-1} · 70 kg^{-1} STPD)	0.81	0.34
Minute volume (L · min^{-1} · 70 kg^{-1} BTPS)	25.5	12.06
Tidal volume (1/70 kg BTPS)	1.11	0.64
Respiratory frequency (breaths/min)	24.71	19.14
Dead space (physiologic)	0.32	0.37
pH	7.32	7.37
Bicarbonate (mmol/L)	21.5	22.7

All variables differed statistically significantly. Other measured variables, including respiratory quotient, arterial oxygen and carbon dioxide tensions, and alveolar-to-arterial gradients, were normal. (Modified with permission of the International Anesthesia Research Society from Macintyre PE, Pavlin EG, Dwersteg JF: Effect of meperidine on oxygen consumption, carbon dioxide production, and respiratory gas exchange in postanesthesia shivering. Anesth Analg 66:751–755, 1987.)

Therefore, anesthetics depress metabolism, but not necessarily to a level less than that during normal sleep. Even barbiturate coma does not depress whole body oxygen consumption.[15] In dogs in barbiturate coma for up to 24 hours, overall oxygen consumption increased by about 12% during the first 24 hours; the greatest consumption occurred in splanchnic and muscle beds, but the greatest relative increase in consumption occurred in the brain and kidneys.

REFERENCES

1. Kennealy JA, Penovich PE, Moore-Nease SE: EEG and spectral analysis in acute hyperventilation. Electroencephalogr Clin Neurophysiol 63:98–106, 1986
2. DiMauro S, Bonilla E, Lee CP, et al: Luft's disease: Further biochemical and ultrastructural studies of skeletal muscle in the second case. J Neurol Sci 27:217, 1976
3. Robin ED, Lewiston NJ, Theodore J, et al: Alveolar hypoventilation caused by "Vera's disease" (thoracic and abdominal muscle contracture)—a new disorder? Cal Med 116:4–35, 1972
4. Jeffrey SW, Smith MJH: Some effects of salicylate on mitochondria from rat liver. Biochemistry 72:462, 1959
5. Shapira Y, Cederbaum SDD, Cancilla PA, et al: Familial polidystrophy, mitochondrial myopathy, and lactate acidemia. Neurology 25:614, 1975
6. Harrison GG: Porcine malignant hyperthermia—the saga of the "hot" pig, in Britt BA (ed): Malignant Hyperthermia. Boston, Martinus Nijhoff, 1987, pp 103–136

7. Sinatra F, Yoshida T, Applebaum M, et al: Abnormalities of carbamyl phosphate synthetase and ornithine transcarbamylase in liver of patients with Reye's syndrome. Pediatr Res 9:829, 1975
8. Haber E, Slater EE: High blood pressure. Sci Am Med 7:17, 1986
9. Askanazi J, Rosenbaum SH, Hyman AI, et al: Respiratory changes induced by the large glucose loads of total parenteral nutrition. JAMA 243:1444, 1980
10. Whipp J, Wasserman K: Effect of anaerobiosis on the kinetics of O_2 uptake during exercise. Fed Proc 45:2942–2947, 1986
11. Wilmore DW: Metabolic Management of the Critically Ill. New York, Plenum, 1977
12. Hagerdal M, Caldwell CB, Gross JB: Intraoperative fluid management influences carbon dioxide production and respiratory quotient. Anesthesiology 59:48–50, 1983
13. Macintyre PE, Pavlin EG, Dwersteg JF: Effect of meperidine on oxygen consumption, carbon dioxide production, and respiratory gas exchange in postanesthesia shivering. Anesth Analg 66:751–755, 1987
14. Mikat M, Peters J, Zindler M, et al: Whole body oxygen consumption in awake, sleeping and anesthetized dogs. Anesthesiology 60:220–227, 1984
15. Gronert GA, Michenfelder JD, Steen PA, et al: Canine whole body and organ system tolerance during 24 hours deep pentobarbital anesthesia. Anesthesiology 58:18–24, 1983

Chapter 6

Transport of Carbon Dioxide

DIFFUSION

If humans were flat like a pancake, the transport of carbon dioxide would not be elaborate; the gas could simply diffuse through the two sides of the pancake and that would be that. Although humans are no pancakes (not withstanding occasional impressions to the contrary), some gas does simply diffuse through the skin where carbon dioxide can be measured with a transcutaneous carbon dioxide analyzer. Cells that lie to the center of our bodies cannot rid themselves so easily of the gas; instead, a complex system serves to transport and eliminate the gas that diffuses through the interstitial space that surrounds the cells where carbon dioxide is produced.

The partial pressure of carbon dioxide (PCO_2) in interstitial fluid surrounding cells closely mirrors that inside the cell because gas can move so easily from one compartment to the other. In either case, PCO_2 normally lies close to 46 mm Hg. Venous blood leaving the capillaries bathing the interstitial areas, therefore, also has a PCO_2 of about 46 mm Hg. When arterial blood with a PCO_2 of 40 mm Hg returns to the interstitial space and the cells, they cannot have a PCO_2 less than 40 mm Hg unless the arterial PCO_2 has been lowered by hyperventilation. The small gradient from the intracellular 46 mm Hg to the arterial 40 mm Hg suffices to draw carbon dioxide from cell to blood via the interstitial fluid (Figure 6.1).

CIRCULATION

Some carbon dioxide travels as dissolved gas in plasma. For every mm Hg of carbon dioxide, plasma accepts 0.65 ml of carbon dioxide gas in solution. At partial pressures of 40 or 46 mm Hg, 1 L of plasma, therefore, can accommodate about 26 to 30 ml of carbon dioxide gas. This is based on the assumption that body temperature is 37°C because temperature affects the solubility of gases in liquids. The solubility of carbon dioxide gas at 44°C is much lower than at 20° C. The relationship is exponential; several other factors, which are also

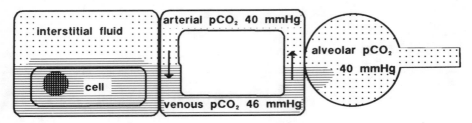

FIGURE 6.1   *Gradients of carbon dioxide tension. The diagram depicts the concentration gradient of carbon dioxide tension (PCO₂) from interstitial fluid and cell to venous blood to alveolus and from there to arterial blood. Interstitial fluid equilibrates with arterial and cellular PCO₂. Interstitial PCO₂ can decrease if arterial PCO₂ decreases.*

temperature-sensitive, influence the amount of carbon dioxide transported in blood.

If dissolved carbon dioxide were the only means of transporting it, if 300 ml/min were produced (at rest), and if all carbon dioxide could be eliminated in the lungs as blood passes by the alveoli, an abnormally high cardiac output of 10 L/min (each liter delivering 30 ml of carbon dioxide to the lungs) would be needed to expel metabolically produced carbon dioxide from the body. Further, during exercise or shivering when carbon dioxide production is doubled or tripled, cardiac output could not keep pace. Thus, the body cannot depend solely on the transport of dissolved gas to the lungs; other mechanisms must be available. The power of these other mechanisms is illustrated by the fact that, during one pass through the lungs, PCO₂ decreases from about 46 mm Hg on the venous side (mixed venous blood and blood in the pulmonary artery) to only 40 mm Hg on the arterial side (pulmonary vein and the systemic arteries beyond), just as PCO₂ increases by only about 6 mm Hg (from 40 to 46 mm Hg) during its sojourn through the capillaries linking the arterioles to the venules (Figure 6.1).

We can look at this extraordinary feat of gas transport in yet another way. If the only mechanism for eliminating carbon dioxide from the body were the transport of dissolved gas transported to the lungs, and if PCO₂ decreased from 46 to 40 mm Hg during one passage through the lungs, a normal cardiac output (approximately 5 L/min) would enable in 1 min exhalation of only 19.5 ml of carbon dioxide (0.65 ml of carbon dioxide per mm Hg · 6 mm Hg · 5 L), instead of the 200 ml that actually must be exhaled (at rest).

The enormous capacity of the system that transports carbon dioxide can be demonstrated simply. Take 1 L of venous blood and remove all the carbon dioxide, *e.g.,* by adding acid to the blood. This reveals that 1 L of venous blood (with a PCO₂ of only 46 mm Hg) contains about 530 ml of carbon dioxide. We can easily imagine how the body can deliver 300 ml of carbon dioxide to the lungs with a cardiac output of a few liters per minute. Indeed, much carbon dioxide will have to be carried back again into the arterial blood if we want to eliminate only 300 ml/min with a cardiac output of 4 to 5 L/min. The question is as follows: how can carbon dioxide that is not physically dissolved be carried by the blood? The answer is a fascinating tale.

Transport of Carbon Dioxide in Plasma and Red Blood Cells

Emerging from the cell and entering the interstitial space, plasma, and red blood cells, carbon dioxide encounters water, proteins, and hemoglobin. In water alone, little happens because hydration of carbon dioxide to carbonic acid proceeds slowly, but when carbon dioxide gas enters the red blood cell, the effect is dramatic. First, carbonic anhydrase in the cell enormously accelerates hydration of carbon dioxide to carbonic acid (Figure 6.2). Almost at once some of the carbonic acid dissociates into hydrogen and bicarbonate ions. Hydrogen is bound by buffers, but bicarbonate, a convenient package for about 70% of the carbon dioxide, is carried away in red blood cells. As bicarbonate is generated, ionic equilibrium is maintained within the red blood cell by displacement of the chloride ion from the cell to the plasma, the so-called chloride shift or Hamberger effect.

This important system has another perspective. The PCO_2 is 46 mm Hg in venous blood reaching the right heart and 40 mm Hg in arterial blood leaving the left heart, and those partial pressures must be in equilibrium with the hydrogen buffers and the bicarbonate that enable carbon dioxide elimination. Within this simple statement lie hidden complex relationships between carbon dioxide gas in solutions and carbon dioxide in other forms. The concentration of hydrogen ion, the ratio of reduced hemoglobin to oxyhemoglobin, the function of buffers, the presence of carbonic anhydrase, and the effect of temperature are essential to this relationship.

ACID–BASE BALANCE

Gaseous carbon dioxide produced by the metabolism of substrate and oxygen always forms inside a cell. Any disturbance in carbon dioxide production is an

$$CO_2 + H_2O \overset{\text{carbonic anhydrase}}{\rightleftharpoons} H_2CO_3 \overset{\text{ionic dissociation}}{\rightleftharpoons} H^+ + HCO_3^-$$

FIGURE 6.2 The transformations of carbon dioxide. Carbon dioxide (CO₂) and water (H₂O) can be transformed into hydrogen ions and bicarbonate. When the enzyme carbonic anhydrase is inhibited, as for instance with acetazolamide (Diamox), carbon dioxide in blood increases and bicarbonate formation decreases.

intracellular disturbance, which is sometimes overlooked in clinical discussion because we measure carbon dioxide and pH in blood or plasma or carbon dioxide in gas. A metabolic acidosis or alkalosis always starts as an intracellular process (unless we infuse acids or alkali into a patient's blood). Although carbon dioxide and oxygen can traverse the cell membrane with ease, hydrogen ions cannot. This makes it difficult to conceive a picture of distribution of carbon dioxide and hydrogen ions, for instance, between blood and cerebrospinal fluid, where the blood-brain barrier hinders the free distribution of charged or bulky and nongaseous substances.

Carbon dioxide is vital in the maintenance of acid–base hemostasis; hyperventilation and hypoventilation can lead to respiratory alkalosis or acidosis or can compensate metabolic acid–base disturbances. Because of the interaction of water with carbon dioxide and its conversion into bicarbonate, carbon dioxide also plays a role in biochemical buffering in the body. To appreciate this role, it is necessary to examine the components of the Henderson-Hasselbalch equation, the equation most common in the discussion of acid–base disturbances. This equation is the logarithmic offspring of the nonlogarithmic Henderson equation. The Henderson equation is

$$[H^+] = K \cdot \frac{PCO_2 \cdot 0.031}{\text{bicarbonate}}$$

The logarithmic Henderson-Hasselbalch equation is

$$pH = pK + \log \frac{\text{bicarbonate}}{PCO_2 \cdot 0.031}$$

Both formulas show the interdependence of carbon dioxide, bicarbonate, and hydrogen ion activity. In Henderson's formula a normal hydrogen ion value might be 40 nanomoles (nmol/L), which would be expressed as pH 7.4 according to Henderson-Hasselbalch. With acidemia a pathologically high hydrogen ion concentration might be 80 nmol/L, which translates into a pH of 7.1, whereas 20 nmol/L $[H^+]$/L (corresponding to a pH of 7.7) represents a pathologically low hydrogen ion concentration, as found in severe alkalemia.

Both formulations contain the constant K, which describes the concentration (or activity) of hydrogen ion at which the ratio of carbon dioxide to bicarbonate is unity, or 1. For Henderson's formula, K equals 800, *i.e.*, when there are 800 nmol/L of hydrogen ion in 1 L of blood at 37°C, the concentration of carbon dioxide must equal that of bicarbonate. In the Henderson-Hasselbalch formula, K is converted into

$$\log \frac{1}{K}$$

and is then called pK, just as the pH of the Henderson-Hasselbalch formula equals in Henderson's formulation:

$$\log \frac{1}{[\text{H}^+]}$$

Under normal physiologic conditions, pK equals 6.1. Therefore, if bicarbonate were 10 mmol/L and carbon dioxide were 10 mmol/L, pH would be 6.1. K and pK are treated as constants; however, at abnormal physiologic temperatures and extremes of acidity or alkalinity, pK ceases to be 6.1 and, therefore, is not really a constant. However, for this discussion of physiologic circumstances, we can safely treat pK as a constant and ignore it forthwith.

As we are concerned with carbon dioxide, let us examine how changes in pH or bicarbonate affect carbon dioxide in blood. First we will add hydrogen ions (pH will decrease) either from an external source, such as the infusion of hydrochloric acid, or from an internal source, such as the liberation of lactic acid during hypoxemia. Assume that the patient's trachea is intubated and that ventilation is being mechanically controlled and minute ventilation will not change. Assume also that the patient was in a steady state until acid began to accumulate in blood, whereupon pH decreased from 7.4 to 7.1. Assume that all compensatory processes are suspended long enough for us to observe the process run its course (Figure 6.3).

We can predict that the addition of hydrogen ions (H^+) must cause an imbalance that, in turn, will cause bicarbonate to combine with hydrogen, carbonic acid to form, and carbon dioxide to be liberated. The acid–base formulas (Henderson or Henderson-Hasselbalch) enable us to calculate how much bicarbonate must combine with hydrogen and how much carbon dioxide will be liberated. In essence, the decrease of pH from 7.4 to 7.1 represents a doubling of the concentration of hydrogen ion. If the ratio of bicarbonate to carbon dioxide had been 20:1 at a pH of 7.4, the ratio would be 10:1 at a pH of 7.1. The sum of bicarbonate and carbon dioxide, however, would not have changed under the artificial conditions imposed by us for this discussion. Thus, as long as ventilation is not adjusted, acidic conditions increase PCO_2 in the arterial blood.

The opposite process, withdrawing hydrogen ions, would reduce PCO_2 in blood. Similarly, adding bicarbonate would also influence the right side of the equation (Figure 6.4). In this case, however, the hydrogen ion would be consumed in the formation of carbonic acid. Yet the newly formed carbonic acid would dissociate and, once again, carbon dioxide would be liberated and,

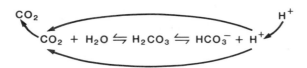

FIGURE 6.3 *Metabolic acidosis. The addition of hydrogen ions leads to the liberation of carbon dioxide (CO_2).*

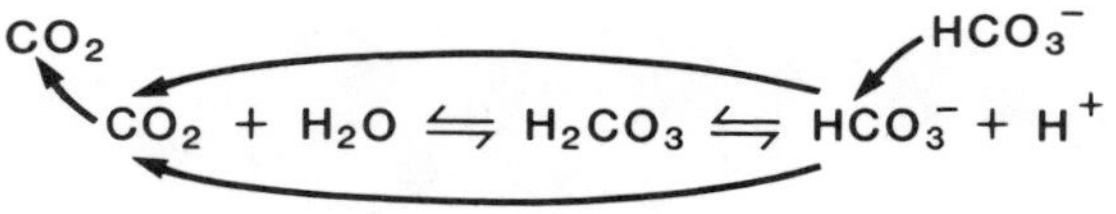

$$CO_2 + H_2O \rightleftharpoons H_2CO_3 \rightleftharpoons HCO_3^- + H^+$$

FIGURE 6.4   *Metabolic alkalosis. The addition of bicarbonate leads to the liberation of carbon dioxide (CO_2).*

again, ventilation would need to be increased to maintain normal levels of carbon dioxide in blood. By the same token, the accumulation of carbon dioxide during hypoventilation will drive the equation in the opposite direction; bicarbonate will increase, as will hydrogen activity. Conversely, hyperventilation will lower PCO_2 in blood, and bicarbonate will be consumed even as pH will increase.

These relationships give rise to the familiar clinical terminology of acidemia and alkalemia that is of either respiratory or metabolic origin. Acidemia and alkalemia refer to changes measured in blood. Acidosis and alkalosis are more general terms used to refer to acid–base imbalances that affect cells and organs.

Chapter 7

Physical Effects on Gas

TEMPERATURE

Temperature affects the volume of a gas as long as pressure remains constant. To estimate the effect of temperature, we assume that carbon dioxide behaves as an ideal gas and we apply the universal gas equation, which is usually written as:

$$PV = 62.36 \text{ n T}$$

where P is pressure in mm Hg, V is volume in liters, n is the quantity of gas in gram mols, and T is the temperature in absolute degrees (273°Kelvin [K] = O°C). Assume that, at a certain pressure and a temperature of 20°C, a quantity of carbon dioxide will have a volume of 250 ml. At the same pressure but at 37°C (an increase in temperature by 17°K), gas will expand by 17/293 times its original volume. Thus, the gas will expand by 17/293 · 0.25, or 14.5 ml, which will occupy 264.5 ml instead of the 250 ml at 20°C. Carbon dioxide is not an ideal gas, but the principle of expansion with increased temperature is applicable.

HUMIDITY

Comparing inspired gases that are bone dry (and at room temperature) with alveolar gases that are saturated with water vapor (and at body temperature) presents difficulties. It is therefore helpful to report all values as if the gas were saturated with water vapor and at body temperature (body temperature and atmospheric pressure completely saturated with water vapor [BTPS]).

Gas entering the respiratory tract through the mouth and nose or endotracheal tube is humidified as it passes through the respiratory passages. The amount of water vapor (percentage in the gas sample or partial pressure) depends on the temperature of the gas, not on the partial pressure of the ambient air or of any other gas present. At 37.1°C, water vapor exerts a pressure of 47 mm Hg, regardless of the barometric pressure (Table 7.1).

The gases delivered through pipelines or from cylinders that are used in anesthesia systems or ventilators are said to be bone dry, devoid of water

Table 7.1   Pressure of Water Vapor at Different Temperatures

Temperature		Vapor Pressure (mm Hg)
°C	°F	
20	68.0	17.4
25	77.0	23.7
26	78.8	25.2
27	80.6	26.7
28	82.4	28.3
29	84.2	30.0
30	86.0	31.5
31	87.8	33.7
32	89.6	35.6
33	91.4	37.7
34	93.2	39.8
35	95.0	41.8
36	96.8	44.2
37	98.6	46.6
38	100.4	49.3
39	102.2	52.0
40	104.0	54.9
41	105.8	58.3
42	107.6	61.5
43	109.4	64.8
44	111.2	68.2

vapor. Assume that a patient at some mountain resort hospital were to inhale a bone-dry gas mixture of 30% oxygen, 68% nitrous oxide, and 2% isoflurane; the barometric pressure would be 647 mm Hg and the dry gas mixture would contain 194 mm Hg of oxygen (30% of 647 mm Hg), 440 mm Hg of nitrous oxide (68% of 647 mm Hg), and 13 mm Hg of isoflurane (2% of 647 mm Hg). Once inhaled, the gases would be humidified and, instead of there being 647 mm Hg available for the three gases (oxygen, nitrous oxide, and isoflurane), there would be only 600 mm Hg (647 mm Hg − 47 mm Hg) because we are assuming a temperature of 37.1°C and complete humidification. Thus, humidification lowers the partial pressure of oxygen (PO_2) from 194 to 180 mm Hg (30% of 600) and that of nitrous oxide and isoflurane from 440 to 408 mm Hg and 13 to 12 mm Hg, respectively. The relationships of oxygen to nitrous oxide and to isoflurane would remain the same (30 to 68 to 2) even though their partial pressures would change.

TEMPERATURE AND HUMIDITY COMBINED

Assume that you have measured the volume of carbon dioxide in expired gas that is saturated with water vapor and at room temperature (ambient temperature and pressure saturated with water vapor [ATPS]). The following formula will serve:

$$\text{Volume of gas in lungs} = \text{volume of exhaled gas} \cdot F$$

where gas in lungs is measured in BTPS and exhaled gas in ATPS. F is calculated as:

$$F = \frac{273 + \text{body temperature}}{273 + \text{room temperature}} \times \frac{P_B - P_{H_2O} \text{ at room temperature}}{P_B - P_{H_2O} \text{ at body temperature}}$$

where P_B is barometric pressure and P_{H_2O} is partial pressure of water vapor.

RESPIRATORY QUOTIENT

Another complicating factor in calculating the volume of alveolar gas is introduced by the simultaneous addition of carbon dioxide to and removal of oxygen from the alveoli. Blood at 46 mm Hg flowing past the alveoli eliminates enough carbon dioxide to bring the partial pressure of carbon dioxide (PCO_2) in the alveoli to 40 mm Hg. At the same time, oxygen is absorbed and mixed venous blood arriving with a PO_2 of 46 mm Hg leaves the alveolus as arterialized blood with a PO_2 of 97 mm Hg. If the respiratory quotient (RQ) were 1.0 for every milliliter of oxygen absorbed, 1 ml of carbon dioxide would be eliminated in the alveoli. More often than not, the RQ does not reach 1.0 and more oxygen is absorbed from the alveoli than carbon dioxide is added to them. The volume of gas in the alveoli thus deflates slightly and the partial pressures in the alveolus adjust.

The alveolar gas equation, commonly used to calculate average PO_2 in the alveoli, takes the RQ into account:

$$P_AO_2 = F_IO_2 \times (713) - P_ACO_2 \times \left[F_IO_2 + \frac{1 - F_IO_2}{RQ} \right]$$

which can be rewritten to solve for PCO_2 in the alveolus as follows:

$$P_ACO_2 = \frac{F_IO_2 \times (713) - P_AO_2}{F_IO_2 + \dfrac{1 - F_IO_2}{RQ}}$$

where F_IO_2 is the fraction of oxygen inhaled and P_AO_2 is the partial pressure of oxygen in the alveoli. Clearly, if RQ = 1.0, *i.e.,* if as much oxygen is absorbed from the alveoli as carbon dioxide is added to them, the RQ is ignored. Instead of 713 (which represents the partial pressure of gas fully saturated with water vapor at an atmospheric pressure of 760 mm Hg and a temperature of 37.1°C), we could write (Patm − P_{H_2O}) to account for different barometric pressures (Patm) and different water vapor pressures at temperatures different from 37.1°C (Table 7.1).

ESTIMATION OF EFFECTIVE ALVEOLAR VENTILATION

The alveolar gas equation simply states that alveolar ventilation affects both the alveolar concentration of carbon dioxide and, assuming that arterial blood reflects alveolar gas, also the arterial PCO_2 in direct proportion. The equation can be rewritten as follows:

$$F_ACO_2 = \frac{\dot{V}_{CO_2}}{\dot{V}_A}$$

where F_ACO_2 is the fraction of carbon dioxide in alveolar gas, $\dot{V}_{CO_2}$ the liters of carbon dioxide produced per minute, and $\dot{V}_A$ the liters of alveolar ventilation per minute, all of which is quite straightforward, for the most part, because we have to discuss alveolar, rather than minute, ventilation. Some of each breath is wasted because a portion of inhaled gas does not participate in gas exchange.

Assume a patient with a respiratory rate of 10 has a minute volume of 6000 ml. Effective alveolar minute ventilation might be 4000 ml (Figure 7.1) with a tidal volume of 600 ml and a physiologic dead space of 200 ml. Let us now double minute volume to 12,000 ml by increasing respiratory rate to 20 breaths/min. Effective alveolar ventilation will have increased from 4000 ml (400 ml × 10 breaths) to 8000 ml (400 ml × 20 breaths). Take the same patient and again double minute ventilation from 6000 to 12,000 ml, this time not by changing respiratory rate but, instead, by doubling tidal volume from 600 to 1200 ml. Assume that dead space ventilation remains the same, *i.e.*, 2000 ml (200 ml × 10 breaths). Alveolar ventilation, however, will have increased from 4000 (400 ml × 10 breaths) to 10,000 ml (1000 × 10 breaths) instead of to only 8000 ml that resulted when we changed the respiratory rate. Thus, it is not simply a matter of doubling minute volume; we have to account for the effective alveolar ventilation.

As we have already seen, the equation for estimating alveolar or arterial PCO_2 also contains a term for alveolar ventilation. We can therefore rearrange the equation and estimate the effective alveolar ventilation from

$$F_ACO_2 = \frac{\dot{V}_{CO_2}}{\dot{V}_A}$$

to

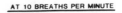

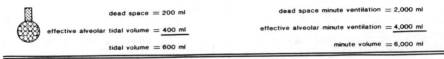

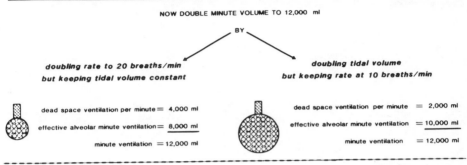

FIGURE 7.1 *Effects on minute volume. Changes in minute volume have different effects on effective alveolar ventilation depending on whether tidal volume or respiratory rate is adjusted.*

$$\dot{V}_A = \frac{\dot{V}_{CO_2}}{F_ACO_2}$$

An example would be a patient with an alveolar FCO_2 (where F is a fraction of any gas, an F of 1 meaning that gas composes 100% of the volume, or an F of 0.05, 5% of volume) of 0.05 and a carbon dioxide production of 300 ml/min. Alveolar ventilation would be estimated as:

$$\dot{V}_A = 0.3/0.05$$

$$\dot{V}_A = 6 \text{ L/min}$$

If we now wish to express the concentration of carbon dioxide in the alveoli not as a fraction or as a percentage but as a partial pressure of all the gases exerting a pressure in the alveoli, we must account for water vapor and correct for body temperature. To do this, we introduce a correction factor of 0.863* and the formula now reads:

---

*When dealing with gases at standard temperature and pressure, dry (STPD), and at body temperature saturated with water vapor (BTPS), conversion factors are used. Here are their derivations:

In the formula,

$$\dot{V}_A = 0.863 \times \frac{\dot{V}_{CO_2}}{P_ACO_2}$$

The effective alveolar ventilation would be 6 L, which would result in an alveolar pCO_2 of 43 mm Hg.

$$\dot{V}_A = \frac{\dot{V}_{CO_2}}{F_ACO_2},$$

$\dot{V}_{CO_2}$ is expressed in STPD. To convert to BTPS, Boyle's law

$$P_1 \times V_1 = P_2 \times V_2$$

and Charles's law

$$\frac{V_1}{V_2} = \frac{T_1}{T_2}$$

are used. Combining the 2 equations yields

$$\frac{P_1 V_1}{T_1} = \frac{P_2 V_2}{T_2}$$

where, for STPD,

$$T_1 = 0\ °C = 273\ °K$$
$$P_1 = 760\ mm\ Hg$$

and for BTPS,

$$T_2 = 37°C = 310°K$$
$$P_2 = 760 - 47 = 713\ mm\ Hg.$$

Rearranging and substituting,

$$V_2 = \frac{P_1 V_1 T_2}{T_1 P_2} = \frac{(760) \times (310)}{(273) \times (760-47)} \times V_1$$
$$V_2 = 1.21\ V_1$$

$$\dot{V}_{A_{BTPS}} = \frac{\dot{V}_{CO_2}\ (STPD)\ (1.21)}{F_ACO_2}$$

To convert F_ACO_2 to P_ACO_2 we multiply the equation by 713 mm Hg, which yields

$$\dot{V}_{A_{BTPS}}\ (ml/min) = \frac{\dot{V}_{CO_2}\ STPD \times 863}{P_ACO_2}$$

Chapter 8

Ventilation-to-Perfusion Ratio

NORMAL RATIO

The lung, that spectacular organ where air and water meet, brings blood (without danger of drying it) into juxtaposition with gas and, thus, links two extraordinary processes. One, ventilation, brings into the body and humidifies fresh gas and removes the gaseous by-product, carbon dioxide. Even though ventilation occurs in breaths rather than a continuous wind, gas exchange is practically continuous. This is true because each breath draws a tidal volume of gas, about 500 ml, into a large reservoir of about 2300 ml, the functional residual capacity (FRC), which minimizes fluctuations in gaseous components in the alveoli. Imagine 500 ml of carbon dioxide-free gas being blown into a bag holding 2300 ml of gas containing 5% carbon dioxide; the concentration of carbon dioxide in the resulting 2800 ml of gas would drop only to about 4.1% (and only if the gases were completely mixed within one breath). Because blood constantly delivers more carbon dioxide to the lungs, the expired tidal volume contains about 5% carbon dioxide. Thus, every breath removes only about 5% of 500 ml of carbon dioxide, or 25 ml. In 10 breaths, that adds up to about 250 ml, enough to wash out the carbon dioxide produced in 1 min by a resting adult. Slight fluctuations in alveolar carbon dioxide concentrations caused by breathing is not measured clinically, yet must affect the level of carbon dioxide in pulmonary venous blood. Current technology does not enable us to measure the small fluctuations in gas concentrations imposed by ventilation, a cycle that occurs in a matter of seconds. At about 70 beats/min, the heart pushes blood through a long pulmonary capillary bed, but blood flows practically in a steady stream because the branching of an ever-widening system of ever-narrowing lumens dampens the fluctuations in pressure and flow.

    The dark blood of the pulmonary artery arrives at the alveoli with about 46 mm Hg of carbon dioxide, and while it becomes arterialized drops the partial pressure (PCO_2) to 40 mm Hg. Inspired air normally contains no carbon dioxide (actually about 0.03%, not enough to concern us here) and about 21% oxygen; expired air leaving the patient's airway is laden with about 5% carbon dioxide and only about 16% oxygen. Ideally, ventilation and perfusion should match exactly so that the capacity of one process, ventilation or perfusion, corresponds to the capacity of the other in both directions, into and out of cell, alveolus, lung, or body. This phenomenon, accomplished to an astonishing degree in healthy persons, is described as the ventilation-to-perfusion ratio ($\dot{V}/\dot{Q}$) which ideally equals 1. This ideal match is attained in a compromise in that some areas of the lung are ventilated better than they are perfused (the upper fields), whereas others are perfused better than ventilated (the lower areas).[1] This has to do with gravity rather than anatomy; therefore, position will influence which areas are better perfused. The lung also can call in a number of regulatory tricks by which it can funnel more or less perfusion into one area or the other. For instance, hypoxic blood emerging from one area of the lung would suggest that gas exchange lags behind and that to shunt more blood through that segment would be counterproductive. The healthy lung can throttle blood supply to that area and thus minimize the undesirable consequences of poorly oxygenated blood circulating on the arterial side. This so-called hypoxic pulmonary vasoconstriction operates to great advantage in conditions in which blood flow and ventilation are poorly matched, as, for instance, when the chest has been opened, when position is changed from supine to lateral, when mechanical ventilation disturbs the match of ventilation to perfusion observed during spontaneous ventilation, when the surgeon compresses a lung, or when something interferes with ventilation to a segment of the lungs. Hypoxic pulmonary vasoconstriction cannot correct all shortcomings of ventilation-to-perfusion matching, and this mechanism can be suppressed by anesthesia. Then the full impact of mismatching becomes apparent. Hypoxic pulmonary vasoconstriction, therefore, to a greater or lesser degree, maintains the ventilation-to-perfusion relationship as close to 1 as possible, and this is important not only to oxygen but also to carbon dioxide.

It is impossible to detect mismatched $\dot{V}/\dot{Q}$ by capnography. Instead, we must compare the expired with the arterial concentration of carbon dioxide (Figure 8.1). The expired gas leaving the mouth late during exhalation is thought to represent the alveolar partial pressure of carbon dioxide (P_ACO_2). The question remains whether end-expired gas (P_ECO_2) is truly alveolar (P_ACO_2).

The expired carbon dioxide concentration may be expressed as a relative term in percent or as partial pressure in mm Hg or K Pa. Normal values for percent peak expiratory carbon dioxide lie between 5% and 6%, which equals a P_ECO_2 of 36 to 44 mm Hg or 4.78 to 5.85 K Pa. Calculating partial pressure from percentage must take into account that water vapor in the alveoli (47 mm Hg at 37.1°C body temperature) occupies volume; assuming a barometric pressure of 760 mm Hg, only 713 mm Hg (760 − 47) are available for gases other than water vapor. (See inside back cover for a conversion table of mm Hg into kPa.)

When ventilation and perfusion are well matched, the gradient between $PaCO_2$ and P_ECO_2 is small. With anesthesia and mechanical ventilation, the gradient increases little, in healthy subjects to 4 to 5 mm Hg owing to small inequities in addition to physiologic shunts.

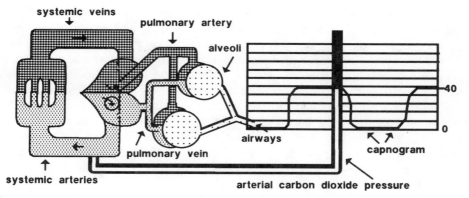

FIGURE 8.1 *Normal ventilation/perfusion. In this diagram of the systemic and pulmonary circulation, two well-perfused and well-ventilated alveoli represent the lungs. With ventilation, carbon dioxide concentration (pCO_2) rises and falls in the trachea. Expired concentrations (P_ECO_2) are recorded as a capnogram (far right). A manometer (dark vertical column) tapping the systemic artery shows the carbon dioxide tension in arterial blood ($PaCO_2$). Superimposing $PaCO_2$ on the expired capnogram (P_ECO_2) depicts the relationship between these two values; in this example with normal values, P_ECO_2 and $PaCO_2$ are practically identical.*

Because blood brings carbon dioxide to the lungs and the lungs expel it, the gradient of carbon dioxide should decrease from blood to alveoli. Occasionally, however, this relationship is reversed, and P_ECO_2 exceeds $PaCO_2$. Such a gradient, if not caused by artificial measurement, is difficult to explain.[2] A greater frequency of reversed gradient (the expired carbon dioxide tension being greater than the arterial) has been reported with some clinical conditions, *e.g.*, in women during Cesarean section,[3] than with others. Also, such a negative gradient is reportedly more common with large than with small tidal volumes[4] and with reduced FRC.

ABNORMAL RATIO

In this discussion, we do not address reflexes that regulate blood flow to different segments of the lung. We are only interested in the broad principles of how the $\dot{V}/\dot{Q}$ ratio can vary.

Causes of Decreased Ratio

When a bronchus is blocked and ventilation of a pulmonary segment is prevented but perfusion of that segment continues, the concentration gradient from alveolus to artery increases (Figure 8.2). Assume that all was well before the obstruction and that the patient's normal alveolar and arterial concentrations of carbon dioxide were in a steady state. Now a block occurs. It could have been caused by mucus or aspirated vomitus, by an endotracheal tube that slipped into a mainstem bronchus (leaving the other lung without ventilation) or that occluded the right upper lobe bronchus, or by a surgical intervention. Without an adjustment in ventilatory pattern, more gas would ventilate the unobstructed parts of the lungs, which may eliminate more carbon dioxide than before. The area that is perfused and not ventilated sends (shunts) mixed venous blood into the pulmonary vein. Therefore, the $PaCO_2$ increases and so does the arterial-to-alveolar gradient. (We discuss this problem later in relation to asthma.)

As the condition persists, complex mechanisms begin to operate. The increasing $PaCO_2$ eventually leads to higher levels of carbon dioxide in venous blood. More carbon dioxide, thus, can be removed with every breath from the perfused and well-ventilated area. Also, more carbon dioxide is added by the blood shunted past the nonventilated segment. Of greater clinical concern is the hypoxemia that is likely to develop under such conditions. Therefore, the arterial-to-alveolar gradient for oxygen should always be monitored as well as the carbon dioxide. This type of $\dot{V}/\dot{Q}$ mismatch is often referred to as a shunt. There are two types of shunts: an anatomic shunt, in which vessels simply bypass the alveolar tissue, and a capillary shunt, in which blood traverses alveolar tissue but fails either to absorb oxygen or to release carbon dioxide or in which gas exchange itself is badly impaired.

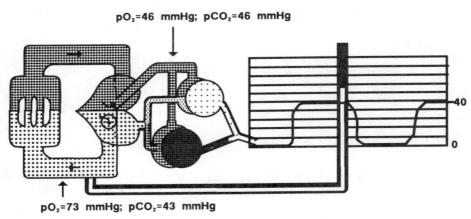

pO_2=46 mmHg; pCO_2=46 mmHg

pO_2=73 mmHg; pCO_2=43 mmHg

FIGURE 8.2   *Ventilation/perfusion mismatch caused by an occluded airway. A part of the lung deprived of ventilation (dark airway and alveolus) is perfused normally but cannot exchange gas. Carbon dioxide-containing blood gets carried into the pulmonary vein and from there into the systemic circulation. The gradient between end-tidal (P_ECO_2) to carbon dioxide tension ($PaCO_2$) rises because the removal of CO_2 from the well-ventilated lung progresses while arterial PCO_2 rises.*

Anatomic Shunt

With an anatomic shunt (Figure 8.3) ventilation appears well matched to perfusion of the alveoli, but part of the right ventricular output bypasses the lung (*e.g.*, as with a congenital cardiac defect associated with a right-to-left shunt). The consequence is the same as with airway obstruction in that mixed venous blood will arrive in the left atrium. The gradient of arterial-to-alveolar PCO_2 will be larger than normal.

Causes of Increased Ratio

Ventilation-to-perfusion mismatch can be caused by pulmonary embolism,[5] whether from blood clot, air, fat, or tumor (Figure 8.4). Also, during anesthesia and operation, constriction or compression of pulmonary vessels or a loss in fine regulation of blood flow may cause mismatched ventilation; this latter cause of mismatch has also been reported in patients in shock.

Ventilation-to-perfusion inequalities often occur in many small segments in which the degrees of $\dot{V}/\dot{Q}$ mismatch vary. To picture the consequences of such a mismatch, assume that a patient's lungs had been well ventilated, that the arterial PCO_2 had been steady at 36 mm Hg, and that peak expired PCO_2 had been 40 mm Hg. Now several small emboli are flung into the pulmonary artery. Suddenly, several areas of the lung are no longer perfused but are still well ventilated. The blood in the lungs distal to the clot still contains carbon dioxide. As other parts of the lungs are ventilated, this stagnant carbon dioxide will be washed out, the amount of which will depend on the quantity of blood that has been cut off from the circulation. In this situation recording a cap-

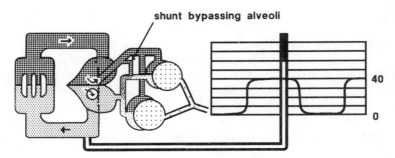

shunt bypassing alveoli

40

0

FIGURE 8.3 *The shunt. The lung is normally ventilated, but a shunt (either intra-cardiac or pulmonary) enables mixed venous blood, without having exchanged gas, to bypass the lung and reach the pulmonary vein and hence the systemic arterial circulation. Arterial carbon dioxide tension will increase, but the end-tidal concentration may well be normal. The gradient from arterial to end-tidal carbon dioxide tension will be greater than normal.*

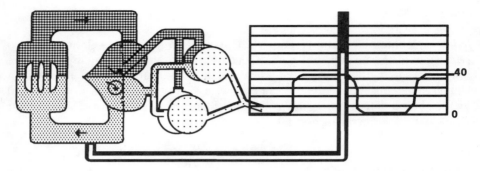

FIGURE 8.4   *Abnormal alveolar dead space. The perfusion of one respiratory unit is blocked, possibly by an embolus, but the unit continues to be well ventilated. Thus, ventilation will be excessive for the amount of carbon dioxide delivered, and the end-tidal tension of carbon dioxide will be lower than the arterial tension, even though neither is necessarily absolutely high.*

nogram on slowly moving paper will generate a typical pattern, an exponentially decreasing level of peak expiratory carbon dioxide (see Figure 1.3).

Once the washout is complete and if no reflexes or other stimuli besides vascular occlusion were to affect perfusion and ventilation, gas ventilating the unperfused lung segments would return from the alveoli without having absorbed carbon dioxide (nor having delivered oxygen). This carbon dioxide-free gas would mix with the carbon dioxide-rich gas returning from well-perfused areas of the lungs. In this situation a capnogram will show low carbon dioxide values after the embolism.

With regard to the arterial side, if total pulmonary blood flow after embolism remains as it was before embolism, the ventilated and perfused areas of the lung will have more perfusion but the same amount of ventilation than before the embolism. If all the extra blood perfusing the ventilated areas cannot release carbon dioxide in the alveoli, arterial PCO_2 will increase. The gradient between $PaCO_2$ and P_ECO_2 will widen. If we increased minute ventilation and removed more carbon dioxide from the ventilated and perfused area, $PaCO_2$ would decrease, but this would have no effect on the abnormally large gradient between $PaCO_2$ and P_ECO_2 because the larger minute ventilation would also increase ventilation of the unperfused area. Often, cardiac output will decrease not only secondary to reflexes, but also, particularly with larger pulmonary emboli, simply because of the obstruction and decreased left atrial and ventricular filling.

The ratio of alveolar to arterial carbon dioxide tension ($P_ACO_2/PaCO_2$ can be used as a rough guideline to estimate the percentage of unperfused but ventilated lung.[6] When the ratio is reduced to about 0.9, about 10% of lung is ventilated but not perfused. With ratios of 0.75 and 0.5, about 40% and 60%, respectively, of the lung is ventilated but not perfused.

In sophisticated experiments numerous measurements can be made to define such details as alveolar ventilation, alveolar dead space, physiologic dead space, airway resistance, carbon dioxide production, flow characteristics, and slope of the capnographic plateau. These measurements, in turn, allow far more detailed analyses of changes in perfusion and ventilation than are attempted here.

$\dot{V}/\dot{Q}$ mismatch is often discussed under the rubric of increased dead space. This can be confusing, however, because mechanical dead space (added by equipment outside the respiratory tract), without impediment to perfusion, increases P_ECO_2. Referring to an increase in the ratio of ventilation (normal) to perfusion (reduced) of the lungs as a $\dot{V}/\dot{Q}$ *mismatch* leaves no doubt about the origin of the disturbance. The term *increased alveolar dead space* would also signal $\dot{V}/\dot{Q}$ mismatch as long as perfusion did not match the increased dead space.

Partially Obstructed Airway

As long as all airways are equally patent, all segments of the lungs cycle respiratory gases in harmony. Often, however, because of asthma or broncho-constriction from other reasons, some areas of the lung empty before others and in extreme situations exhalation is prolonged. This typically leads to a capnogram with a sloping plateau (Figure 8.5; see also Figures 2.9 and 2.10), which depicts the slow emptying of part of the lung at the end of a narrowed airway. Gas exchange in that segment of the lung will be less than optimal because blood flowing to that segment cannot deliver carbon dioxide or absorb oxygen in normal quantities; the arterial blood will have carbon dioxide levels higher than is true for peak expiratory values. The clinician, however, may worry more about oxygenation than carbon dioxide.

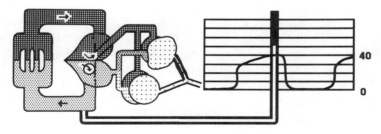

FIGURE 8.5 *The partially obstructed airway. One bronchus is partially obstructed as might be seen with asthma. The alveoli empty unevenly and part of the lung is poorly ventilated but well perfused. An increased gradient of arterial to end-tidal carbon dioxide tension results in a typical sloped plateau of the capnogram. As long as the plateau of the capnogram continues to rise, expiration continues; arterial values can therefore become significantly higher than end-tidal values of carbon dioxide tension.*

PULMONARY DISEASES

Ventilation-to-perfusion abnormalities are well represented in patients treated with intermittent mandatory ventilation; these patients with lung diseases can breathe spontaneously but are given occasional deep breaths to maintain normal oxygenation and to eliminate carbon dioxide. In such patients the peak expired concentration of carbon dioxide has been observed to vary greatly from breath to breath and the gradient from peak expired to arterial carbon dioxide concentration to fluctuate equally widely.[7] It is therefore best not to depend on a single reading but instead to watch the expiratory values over time and use the highest carbon dioxide value that occurs; it will best reflect arterial values. In general, peak expired values will better represent arterial concentrations after a large tidal volume from a spontaneous breath than after an equally large tidal volume from a ventilator breath.[7] Finally, when the peak expiratory value does not truly reflect the concentration of carbon dioxide in alveolar gas, a smart push on the patient's chest often expels a little extra carbon dioxide, which produces a bump on the plateau of the capnogram (see also Figure 2.7).

Abnormalities of $\dot{V}/\dot{Q}$ reflected in the capnogram occur in different combinations in a number of lung diseases. The following descriptions are used to illustrate the relevant principles and are thus simplifications of clinical realities rather than a discussion of the pathophysiology of lung diseases.

Chronic Obstructive Pulmonary Disease

Chronic obstructive pulmonary disease (COPD) consists of several concomitant abnormalities, such as partial obstruction, underventilation of perfused areas, and ventilation of poorly perfused areas, that produce carbon dioxide retention and hypoxemia. Functional residual capacity often increases because of chronic hyperinflation of the lungs (emphysema). Peak expiratory carbon dioxide tensions are also high, but arterial levels are usually even higher, significantly so. Isolated end-tidal samples often are not meaningfully representative because constricted airways and loss of elasticity make emptying the lungs difficult. Indeed, spontaneous exhalation may not have run its slow course and, thus, not reached an expiratory plateau before the next inspiration interrupts the plateau of the capnogram.

Asthma

In this common chronic lung disease, which afflicts approximately 2.5% of the population, reversible bronchoconstriction is the primary abnormality. In an advanced condition inflammation, edema, and air trapping with overdistention of parts of the lung occur. Mucous plugs obstructing the airways complicate the picture. Interference with gas exchange accompanies acute attacks and chronic conditions. There are four grades of asthma that illuminate the results of ventilation abnormalities (Table 8.1). In grade 1 gas exchange is normal even though there is some wheezing.

We can appreciate why PaO_2 decreases as the disease advances. Why carbon dioxide is low in grade 2 and normal in grade 3 and jumps to high only in grade 4 is more complicated. The normal large gradient in oxygen concentration from arterial blood-to-alveolus ($\sim$ 54 mm Hg), as compared with the normal, small gradient for carbon dioxide concentration ($\sim$ 6 mm Hg), sets the stage (Figure 8.6, *top*). Assume that exactly one-half the lung were obstructed and that blood flow were unaffected (Figure 8.6, *bottom*); one-half of the blood draining into the main pulmonary vein will have a PO_2 of 46 mm Hg and a PCO_2 of 46 mm Hg. The ventilated segment will deliver blood with a PO_2 of 100 mm Hg and a PCO_2 of 40 mm Hg into the common pulmonary vein. The resultant mixed blood will thus have a PO_2 of 73 mm Hg ([100 + 46]/2), whereas the $PaCO_2$ will be much less affected, *i.e.*, 43 mm Hg ([46 + 40]/2). This simplified scheme ignores the nonlinear hemoglobin dissociation.

Assume now that, in response to either respiratory reflexes or a sense of dyspnea and because of altered blood gases, the respiratory center induces hyperventilation of ventilated segments of lung. Hyperventilation could easily lower $PaCO_2$ but could not easily restore PaO_2 to normal; with vigorous ventilation $PaCO_2$ can become lower than normal.

We can use the alveolar gas equation to estimate how much additional ventilation of aerated lung would be needed to correct $PaCO_2$, *e.g.*, to lower it from 43 to 40 mm Hg. We would have to decrease the PCO_2 of blood draining the ventilated lung to 37 mm Hg. Were this blood to mix with blood from the unventilated segment ($PvCO_2$ of 46 mm Hg), the mixed blood would have a $PaCO_2$ of 40 mm Hg. The alveolar gas equation states:

$$\dot{V}_A = \frac{\dot{V}_{CO_2}}{F_A CO_2}$$

when volume ($\dot{V}$) is measured in liters per minute.

Table 8.1 Grades of Asthma According to Severity

	Arterial Gas Tensions	
Grade of Asthma	*Oxygen*	*Carbon Dioxide*
1 (mild)	Normal	Normal
2	Low	Low
3	Low	Normal
4 (severe)	Low	High

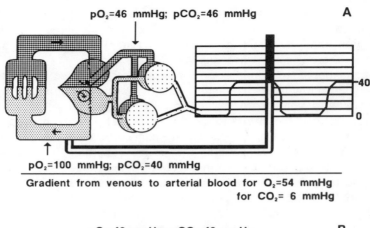

pO₂=46 mmHg; pCO₂=46 mmHg   A

pO₂=100 mmHg; pCO₂=40 mmHg

Gradient from venous to arterial blood for O₂=54 mmHg
for CO₂= 6 mmHg

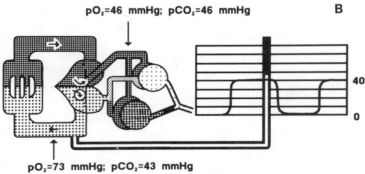

pO₂=46 mmHg; pCO₂=46 mmHg   B

pO₂=73 mmHg; pCO₂=43 mmHg

Gradient from venous to arterial blood for O₂ = 27 mmHg
for CO₂ = 3 mmHg

FIGURE 8.6 *The gradients of partial pressures for carbon dioxide and oxygen. (A) Normally, the concentration gradient from artery to vein is large for oxygen (100 to 46 mm Hg) and small for carbon dioxide (46 to 40 mm Hg). (B) With one lung excluded from ventilation, one-half the blood passes ventilated alveoli, the other does not. Therefore, the arterial values for oxygen and carbon dioxide tensions will be between those of arterial and venous blood. Because the venous-to-arterial partial pressure gradient for oxygen is large and that for carbon dioxide is small, the admixture of venous blood causes a substantial decrease in PaO_2 and only a modest decrease in $PaCO_2$. In this simplified scheme, we have ignored all physiologic consequences of bronchial obstruction.*

Assuming that carbon dioxide production remains constant and that we want to lower expired carbon dioxide from 43 to 37 mm Hg, we would have to increase ventilation by 14%. This estimation assumes ideal conditions, no change in $\dot{V}/\dot{Q}$, and no vascular response to increased ventilation. In patients with advanced disease correction of $\dot{V}/\dot{Q}$ abnormality might be impossible, and neither dyspnea, reflexes, low PaO$_2$, nor high PaCO$_2$ could drive ventilation to keep oxygen and carbon dioxide normal.

Atelectasis

Postoperative atelectasis plagues patients with chronic pulmonary disease who undergo operation. Predisposing factors are advanced age, male gender, obesity, and operations on chest or upper abdomen. The pathophysiology of atelectasis involves the loss of ventilation of a perfused area of the lung. Postoperatively, it is not uncommon to observe tachycardia and a normal or a low peak expiratory PCO$_2$ but normal or high PaCO$_2$ and low PaO$_2$. The abnormal gas values can be explained by the same mechanism outlined for asthma.

INCREASED EXTERNAL DEAD SPACE

In contrast to the increased alveolar dead space caused by occlusion of a pulmonary artery, anatomic dead space can be increased unphysiologically by equipment (Figure 8.7); this is a simple situation. During normal exhalation a certain volume of carbon dioxide-laden air remains in the airways. Added mechanical dead space increases the amount of carbon dioxide-rich gas that must be re-inhaled, which impedes carbon dioxide elimination. A capnogram will show high peak expiratory values. The gradient between arterial and alveolar carbon dioxide tensions should not be affected. Increasing alveolar ventilation can compensate for such increased external dead space, although there are limits to which ventilation can be increased. Some anesthesia systems

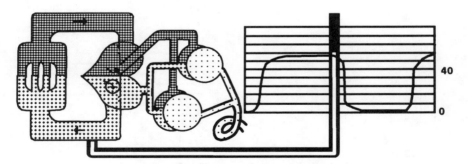

FIGURE 8.7   *Increased mechanical dead space. Dead space was added outside the respiratory system (looped tube), and alveolar dead space was not affected. Carbon dioxide concentrations in expired gas and arterial blood may rise, but the gradient of arterial to end-tidal carbon dioxide tension is normal as long as tidal volume is adequate.*

court such increased equipment dead space. (See also "Dead Space" in Chapter 1.)

SHALLOW VENTILATION

We have repeatedly noted that peak expired concentrations of carbon dioxide depend on the circumstances of ventilation. A tidal volume delivered by mechanical ventilation to a paralyzed patient is less likely to raise carbon dioxide from the depth of the furthest alveolus than is a deep spontaneous breath of equal tidal volume. The smaller the tidal volume, the less likely that peak expired concentrations of carbon dioxide will mirror $PaCO_2$. It is not wise to suspect hyperventilation every time peak expired concentration of carbon dioxide is low. Perhaps the tidal volume is simply too small to raise carbon dioxide from the depth of the lungs (Figure 8.8). Very small tidal volumes might ventilate only dead space, and result in high arterial PCO_2 and concurrent hypoxemia unless respiratory rates are sufficiently high.

COMBINED MECHANISMS

More often than not the clinician encounters complex problems not readily explained by one single mechanism, making an analysis exceedingly difficult. Here, for example, is the story of a 2-year-old child with pulmonary artery stenosis and ventricular septal defect (generating a shunt). During the thoracotomy the surgeon had compressed the right lung (compromising ventilation) in order to complete an anastomosis of the right pulmonary artery to the right subclavian artery, keeping both vessels clamped (compromising perfusion), while suturing the vessels. After completion of the anastomosis, and just before unclamping the vessels, the PaO_2 was 34 mm Hg, and the $PaCO_2$ was 58 mm Hg, while the $PeCO_2$ was only 25.4 mm Hg (Figure 8.9A). The horizontal

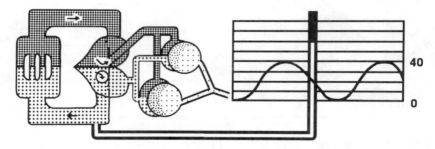

FIGURE 8.8 *Small tidal volume. With small tidal volume the true alveolar carbon dioxide tension may not be reflected in the end-tidal gas, and low peak expired carbon dioxide levels will fail to reveal the high carbon dioxide levels in arterial blood.*

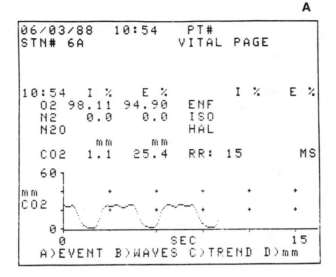

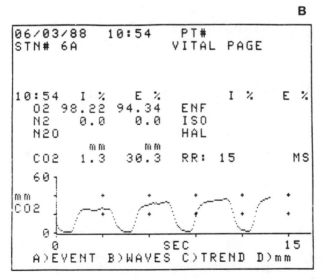

FIGURE 8.9   *Capnograms during thoracotomy. A 2-year-old child with pulmonary artery stenosis and ventricular septal defect who underwent anastomosis of the right subclavian artery to the right pulmonary artery. (A) Right lung compressed. Subclavian and pulmonary artery clamped. $PaCO_2$ is 58 mm Hg. (B) Immediately after unclamping the vessels. (C) One minute later. (D) Two minutes after unclamping. The $PaCO_2$ is now 38 mm Hg.*

C

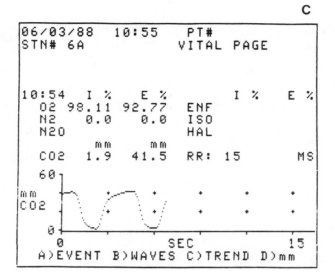

D

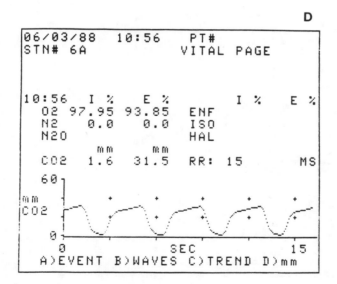

Figure 8.9   *(Continued)*

plateau of the capnogram did not reveal impaired ventilation or slow emptying of the lungs. The capnogram gave evidence of neither the large arterial to end-tidal gradient for PCO_2 nor the poor oxygenation. The pulse oximeter reported 42% saturation. Next, the surgeon unclamped the vessels (Figure 8.9B). The reestablished perfusion of the lungs was reflected in the rising concentrations of carbon dioxide with successive breaths. The plateau became sloped, indicating slow emptying of parts of the lungs. Within 2 minutes, the end-tidal carbon dioxide values increased from 30.3 mm Hg to 41.5 mm Hg (Figure 8.9C), and then fell to 31.5 mm Hg (Figure 8.9D). At this point, the $PaCO_2$ was 38 mm Hg. The PO_2 had also risen to 71 mm Hg, still revealing a large shunt. Pulse oximeter values had also improved, reflecting a saturation of 93%. Thus, in the course of 2 minutes, changes in alveolar dead space and perfusion had generated a roller coaster pattern of arterial and end-tidal carbon dioxide concentrations, even though neither the ventilator nor the fresh gas flows had been adjusted while perfusion and ventilation had been changed.

REFERENCES

1. West JB (ed): Ventilation-Blood Flow and Gas Exchange, ed 2. Oxford, JB Lippincott, 1970
2. Robertson HT, Hlastala MP: Elevated alveolar PCO_2 relative to predicted values during normal gas exchange. J Appl Physiol: Respirat Environ Exercise Physiol 43:357–364, 1977
3. Shankar KB, Moseley H, Kumar Y, et al: Arterial to end-tidal carbon dioxide tension difference during Caesarean section anaesthesia. Anaesthesia 41:698–702, 1986
4. Fletcher R, Jonson B: Deadspace and the single breath test for carbon dioxide during anaesthesia and artificial ventilation. Br J Anaesth 56:109–119, 1984
5. Hatle L, Rokseth R: The arterial to end-expiratory carbon dioxide tension gradient in acute pulmonary embolism and other cardiopulmonary diseases. Chest 66:352–357, 1974
6. Warwick WJ: The end-expiratory to arterial carbon dioxide tension ratio in acute pulmonary embolism. Chest 68:609–611, 1975
7. Weinger MB, Brimm JE: End-tidal carbon dioxide as a measure of arterial carbon dioxide during intermittent mandatory ventilation. J Clin Monit 3:73–79, 1987

PART III

Technologic Perspectives on Capnography

Chapter 9

Capnometry

Few molecules are as critically important to humans as is carbon dioxide. Because of its role in such essential phenomena as metabolism, photosynthesis, combustion, and environmental temperature, a variety of methods have been developed to detect and quantify it. Carbon dioxide's well-documented physical properties are the key to understanding these analytic techniques. At normal temperatures and pressures carbon dioxide is a colorless, odorless gas. Its concentration in air is so small (0.03%) that air is usually treated as if the partial pressure of carbon dioxide were zero. The carbon dioxide molecule has a molecular weight of 44, is very soluble in polar solvents such as water, and reacts with water to form a weak acid. Also, this molecule is easily fragmented and ionized to form charged species and has both symmetric and asymmetric modes of molecular vibration. There is a remarkable similarity between carbon dioxide and nitrous oxide (Table 9.1). Both deviate from ideal gas law to the same degree, as indicated by their mole volumes of 22.25L instead of the ideal mole volume of 22.4L. Both are very soluble in water, which is an advantage physiologically but a disadvantage with on-line methods of analysis in wet systems where out-gassing of carbon dioxide could be a problem.

Measuring the concentration of carbon dioxide noninvasively in respired gas requires a continuous, fast response and the capacity to distinguish different gases from each other. Thus this technology is very different from that used to measure carbon dioxide in a sample of gas or blood. The technologies that have been developed rely on the asymmetric modes of vibration to enable carbon dioxide to absorb infrared light, the symmetric modes of vibration to enable carbon dioxide to scatter light (Raman), and the capacity of the molecule to be charged by an electron beam, to enable the use of mass spectrometry.

TECHNICAL DEVELOPMENTS

The pioneering contributions of Haldane and Scholander in the analysis of physiologic gases relied on measuring changes in gas volume as a gas sample was tracked through a series of absorption steps. Van Slyke improved accuracy by measuring changes in pressure and made modifications that enabled gases in blood samples to be measured. These techniques provide accurate measure-

Table 9.1 Physical Properties of Carbon Dioxide and Physiologically Related Gases

	Nitrous Oxide	Carbon Dioxide	Oxygen	Nitrogen
Molecular weight	44.013	44.007	32.000	28.016
Normal mole volume	22.25	22.25	22.4	22.4
BP (°C)	−89.5	−78.5	−183	−196
Solubility in water at 20°C	0.63	0.878	0.031	0.0164
Viscosity at 20°C (micropoises)	146	146	200	174
Thermal conductivity at 0°C (joules/sec cm³ $\times 10^4/°C$)	1.51	1.45	2.44	2.43
Specific heat at constant pressure (joules/g°C)	0.892	0.898	—	1.030
Velocity of sound (m/sec at 0°C)	258	260.3	314.84	333.64

Reproduced with permission from Nunn JF: Respiratory measurements in the presence of nitrous oxide. Br J Anaesth 30:254, 1958.

ments but require highly trained personnel. Also, these methods capture only isolated moments in a continuously changing concentration of carbon dioxide during the respiratory cycle.

Another approach uses pH. The reaction between carbon dioxide and water that forms carbonic acid has made pH the basis of colorimetric and electrometric procedures. The latter is used in today's blood gas laboratories. The technique is suitably accurate for clinical purposes and requires minimal instruction, but, again, yields only intermittent values. These principles are also embodied in transcutaneous sensors, which provide information continuously and noninvasively, the disadvantage being a long time constant. The skin must be heated to obtain clinically acceptable time constants, and the monitoring site must be changed frequently to prevent burns.

The light absorption of some indicator dyes and the fluorescent intensity of others, fluorescein for example, depend on pH. These dyes have been used in the development of recently introduced monitoring catheters. Their response, however, is also slow, too slow to provide accurate breath-by-breath analysis.

Of the three techniques used to measure carbon dioxide during ventilation—infrared, mass spectrometry, and Raman—infrared is the oldest and most frequently used. It had its beginnings in the early work of Collier in the United States and Luft in Europe.[1,2] In those days instruments were large and cumbersome, were not very reliable, and required frequent calibration. Today's instruments are considerably different. Advances in infrared technology have made optical benches more compact. Microprocessors have revolutionized data processing, improved filtering techniques, and spawned a host of design innovations, which have improved accuracy, increased reliability, and lowered cost.

More recent techniques are mass spectrometry (1981) and, very recently, Raman scattering.[3] Mass spectrometers are highly automatic and measure not only carbon dioxide and the other physiologic gases, but N_2O and other anesthetic agents as well. Raman scattering promises to combine the lower cost of infrared with the multigas capability of mass spectrometry. The technique is so new that first-generation instruments have just become available. At the same time, infrared monitors have been optimized to include anesthetic gases and mass spectrometers redesigned to lower cost. Each technique, infrared, mass spectrometry, and Raman, can effectively measure carbon dioxide, but the principles on which each is based are quite different.

TECHNICAL SPECIFICATIONS

Certain constraints are imposed by measuring techniques. On the other hand, regardless of any constraints, there are specifications that must be satisfied in order to make the results clinically useful.

Range of Carbon Dioxide

Capnometers for clinical use must be able to detect carbon dioxide in the range of 0% to 10% or 76 mm Hg. An extended range to 100 mm Hg is sometimes useful. End-tidal carbon dioxide greater than that will be rarely encountered (*e.g.,* inadvertent hypoventilation or malignant hyperthermia). The range of carbon dioxide should be the same for inspiration as for end-tidal values, which enables rebreathing to be monitored. If rebreathing is not a consideration, a range of 0 to 15 mm Hg is satisfactory for monitoring during surgical operations.

Accuracy

Accuracy, a measurement of how well a monitor detects the true value, should be at least ± 10% of a reading, or ± 3 mm Hg, whichever is larger, as has been recommended in a recent critical study of commercially available capnometers.[4] This level of accuracy is probably sufficient because most clinical applications of capnography benefit from the detection of trends. However, for a more accurate assessment of gradients or when monitors are changed, an uncertainty of ± 5% is preferred; this is about the level of accuracy of the average $PaCO_2$ measurement.

Precision

Precision is the ability to obtain a similar result with repeated measurement. A change in value should not be due to technique or to instrument instability. Repeated short-term measurements should not vary by more than ± 1 mm Hg when measurements are made with a stable gas source.

Calibration

Stability

Long-term stability is an important criterion and determines the frequency of calibration. Even if calibration is automatic, it requires time and may interrupt monitoring. Indeed, to attain the full benefits of capnography, monitoring must be continuous. Automatic zeroing during the inspiratory phase is particularly troublesome because inspiratory gas occasionally contains carbon dioxide (because of such things as a failed expiratory valve, a saturated carbon dioxide absorber, or channelling). As a practical matter, lengthy procedures for calibration should be required infrequently and brief ones no more than once a day. Most modern infrared capnographs are stable for at least 1 month, and perhaps longer.[4]

Confirmation

There are various techniques by which to confirm the accuracy of end-tidal values when a suspicious or significant change has been noted. An optical filter, a beam occluder, or a sample cell containing carbon dioxide all produce signals that can confirm the operation of the instrument. A sample of known carbon dioxide is the most reliable. When such a sample is not readily available, a clinician's own respiratory gases may serve, although this may not be easy to do or may not be reliable in periods of stress.

Procedures

There are three calibration procedures. The oldest is the periodic use of cylinders of calibrated gases. Although early instruments required calibration hourly, it is needed infrequently for modern infrared instruments. Mass spectrometers are less stable and still require hourly calibration, but it is done automatically. Some infrared capnographs have built-in canisters of calibrated gases that make periodic calibrations more convenient.

Another technique makes use of a cell that contains a calibrated mixture of carbon dioxide and nitrogen. This is particularly appropriate for mainstream capnometers because the sample cell can substitute for the airway adapter and be used either for verification or for calibration. A third simple calibrating procedure applicable to Raman scattering uses room air. This is based on the observation that the relative sensitivity to various gases is fixed. After an initial calibration for each gas, only periodic checks of nitrogen and oxygen are necessary.

Interference

Interference can occur in a number of different ways, depending on the analytic technique used. With infrared, interference occurs when the absorption band of a diluent molecule overlaps the selected band for carbon dioxide (cross-interference). This type of interference is possible with nitrous oxide, which has an absorption band (4.55 μ) very close to that almost always used for carbon dioxide (4.26 μ). Most capnometers today have corrections for nitrous oxide, which can be implemented in several ways. The most satisfactory way is to measure nitrous oxide and correct for it directly, which can be done with several instruments. The influence of nitrous oxide on carbon dioxide is determined empirically and appropriate corrections are made. Another technique related to fractional concentration of expired oxygen assumes that the patient is breathing gas composed of oxygen and nitrous oxide, the small percentage of inhalational anesthetic agent being ignored. By measuring oxygen in the inspired gas, the nitrous oxide is estimated under steady state conditions and an appropriate correction is made. During nonsteady state conditions, however, the correction will be in error.

The third correction strategy is a single correction for the midpoint of the range at which nitrous oxide is usually administered, typically 30% to 70%. When the gas composition is at the extremes of the range, however, this correction introduces an error, usually within 2 to 3 mm Hg.

Anesthetic agents have main absorption bands as follows: halothane 13.95 μ; isoflurane 8.5, 11.06, and 12.95 μ; and enflurane 12.24 μ. All have a common band at 3.3 μ. The interference of these molecules is small. They are present at low concentrations, and their main absorption bands are far removed from the 4.26 μ band for carbon dioxide.

Cross-Interference with Raman Scattering

Interference with this technique is very similar to that with infrared instruments. Instead of overlapping absorption bands in the infrared part of the spectrum causing problems, however, the concern is overlapping wavebands of scattered light in the visible part of the spectrum. In the end interference essentially relates to band pass characteristics of the optical filters and the development of appropriate algorithms to sort out the interference.

Cross-Interference with Mass Spectrometry

Just as overlapping absorption bands can be a problem, so can gas molecules with the same or similar mass. For example, nitrous oxide and carbon dioxide have masses that are almost the same, 44.007 for carbon dioxide and 44.013 for nitrous oxide. Mass spectrometers can be designed to resolve such differences; however, such resolution adds complexity and expense. Fortunately, gas molecules can carry more than one charge and can be fragmented. This opens up other possibilities for their detection. (These are discussed in Chapter 11.)

Pressure Broadening

Pressure broadening, or collision broadening, is easily distinguished from cross-interference. Because of cross-interference, carbon dioxide appears to be present even if it is not. This phenomenon does not occur with pressure broadening. The degree to which the absorption band for carbon dioxide widens as pressure increases depends on the diluent molecules (see Chapter 10). Oxygen, nitrogen, and nitrous oxide all have different effects. These have been studied in a systematic way with either carbon dioxide in oxygen[5] or carbon dioxide in nitrogen[6] as the reference compositions. The influence of these gases on the measurement of carbon dioxide, while relatively similar,[5] is closely related to the band pass of the filter and the spectral response of the detector; consequently, the extent of the influence depends on instrument design. Earlier results indicated that the effect of single-diluent gases was independent of the concentration of carbon dioxide;[5,6] more recent work indicates a complex nonlinear relationship when gases are mixed. The effect of water vapor is small but linear with carbon dioxide. At 33°C, the temperature of expired gas, carbon dioxide would be overestimated by 1.5% with a mainstream capnometer if uncorrected.[7] At lower temperatures (vapor pressures), there is less effect. The pressure broadening influence of anesthetic agents has not been reported. Their concentrations are usually so small that the effect is also probably small.

Response Time

One of the most important technical considerations for capnography is response time. This is a measure of how accurately the capnograph portrays variations in carbon dioxide as the patient breathes. This may be quite different from the accuracy with which the capnometer measures a calibrating gas when flow or time is not a factor. The fidelity with which the monitor follows a changing profile is very important because significant diagnostic information can be obtained from the capnographic waveform. An instrument that does not respond fast enough displays erroneously low end-tidal values and erroneously high inspiratory values and may significantly alter the shape of the waveform itself.

Response time can be divided into two parts, a delay time and a rise time.

Delay Time

Delay time is the time it takes the sample to move from the sampling port to the detector; therefore, this is sometimes called lag or transit time. Delay time depends on flow rate, diameter and length of sampling tube, and sample viscosity. For long sampling tubes such as are used with shared mass spectrometers, delay time can be as long as 10 to 20 sec. For shorter tubes such as are used with sidestream infrared instruments, delay time can be a fraction of a second to several seconds; mainstream systems have no delay time. Sometimes the delay time is a processing delay, on the order of 100 to 150 ms. Such delays are not important in capnography per se but could be very important when carbon dioxide concentration is used with flow values to determine carbon dioxide production. Processing delays are associated with either sidestream or mainstream instruments.

Some shared mass spectrometers have two delay times because the rates of sampling flow and measuring flow are not the same. When gas is sampled, sampling flow occurs at a rate sufficient to enable a 20-sec gas sample to be stored in the sampling line. When gas is measured, flow rate is doubled and the 20-sec sample of gas is analyzed within approximately 7 sec, after which the display is updated. The 7 sec is sometimes called dwell time and is the actual time of delay, that is, when monitoring is continuous, the gas sample arrives at the analyzer 7 sec after being sampled. For those mass spectrometers with dedicated infrared carbon dioxide monitors, the delay will depend on where the infrared sample cell is placed in the mass spectrometer sample line. In general, faster flows, shorter tubes with larger lumens, and lower viscosity result in shorter delay time.

Rise Time

Rise time can be characterized in a number of ways. All relate to the assumption that the 0% to 100% response is exponential and lengthy. In most applications we are not interested in how long it takes to obtain 100% response: 90% or 95% is usually satisfactory (Figure 9.1). By subjecting a measuring system to an instantaneous change, *i.e.,* a change that is very fast compared with the response of the system being measured, we can measure the true response characteristics of the system. This is sometimes referred to as a step change. An equation that describes the response is

$$S(t) = I \left(1 - e^{t/\tau}\right)$$

where $S(t)$ is the signal at time t, I is the instantaneous signal, and τ is the

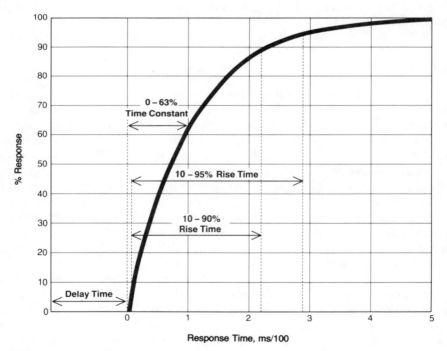

FIGURE 9.1   *For sidestream sampling, response time is equal to the delay or transit time in the sampling catheter plus the measurement rise time. The measurement time constant is defined as the 0 to 63% rise time. Other frequently used rise times are also shown.*

circuit parameter that defines the response. In an electrical circuit, τ would be the product of resistance and capacitance and, in the pulmonary system, of airway resistance and total compliance.

Relative to response time, a system can be uniquely characterized by the value of S when $(t = \tau)$. Knowing that $e = 2.7183$, we can easily show that S $(t = \tau) = 63\%I$. This has been universally adopted as the time constant of a measuring system. Sixty-three percent is still far from what we would like— a 95% or 99% rise time. The difference is easily bridged by multiple time constants; for example 3τ is 95% and 5τ is close to 99%.

Unfortunately, instrument data sheets express response times in different ways (Table 9.2). Most refer to a 10% to 90% response and specify flow rate when appropriate. All rise times can be expressed in terms of an instrument's time constant. For example, if the 10% to 90% rise time is specified as 200 ms, then the time constant is 91 ms (200/2.20). Assuming you wish to make your comparison at 0% to 95% response, or 3τ, the rating would be 273 ms.

What response time is necessary for capnography? The answer to that question has two parts. First, response time must be fast enough to measure both end-tidal and inspiratory carbon dioxide accurately. Second, response time should also be fast enough to provide a high-fidelity display of the carbon dioxide waveform. Interpretation is valid only when the waveform accurately represents the carbon dioxide profile, or at least, accurately enough to detect the events for which the patient is being monitored. No high-frequency changes in waveform of clinical significance have as yet been identified, so an instrument that is responding accurately to clinically encountered breathing rates is satisfactory. The use of time constants to predict performance at various breathing rates is straightforward but should be used only as a guideline because many other factors can have an influence.

If we assume a square wave capnogram (Figure 9.2) (again, the most difficult to follow), an inspiratory-to-expiratory ratio (I:E) of 1:1, and a time constant of 100 ms, we can show that for a 95% response (3τ), one breathing cycle will require 600 ms. Both exhalation and inhalation require 300 ms. If 600 ms are required for one breath, then the instrument can follow 100 breaths/min. Changing circumstances, however, will alter the response. If the I:E ratio

Table 9.2 Time Constant Conversion Table

Specified Rise Time	Time Constant Multiplier
0–50	0.69
0–63	1.00
10–90	2.20
0–90	2.30
10–95	2.89
0–95	3.00
0–99.3	5.00

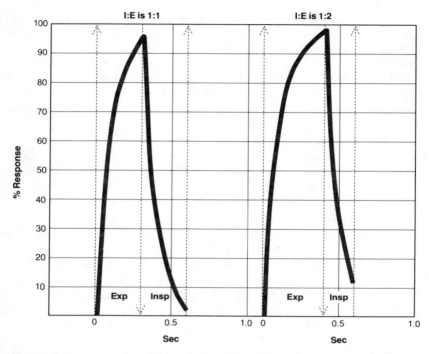

FIGURE 9.2   *The worst case curves demonstrate how rise time and I:E influence capnograms. At a 100 BPM, a rise time of 100 ms will provide both end-tidal and inspiratory carbon dioxide values that will be 5% accurate when the I:E is 1:1. When the I:E is 1:2, the expired carbon dioxide will be within 2% of its final value, but the inspired carbon dioxide will be significantly above its final value. This is nonphysiological as it represents a step change in carbon dioxide.*

changes to 1:2, then at 100 breaths/min, inspiration requires 200 ms and expiration 400 ms. A 98% response will be sensed during expiration (4τ) but only an 86.5% (2τ) during inspiration. This means that the baseline could rise by several mm Hg and, thus, falsely indicate rebreathing. Clinically, however, the changes in concentration are not instantaneous but gradual as faster alveoli mix their contents with slower ones during exhalation. Still, flow could be 30 to 50 L/min during rest and much higher during exercise. Such flow rates occur during periods of rapid changes in carbon dioxide concentration. Consequently, integrating flow with concentration to determine carbon dioxide production is a different problem that requires careful assessment of any time delay between the signals for flow and concentration.

The second part of response time, namely, faithful recording of the capnogram itself, starts with understanding that the shape of the waveform depends in part on where and how gas is measured. Mainstream capnograms may be sharper than sidestream capnograms, but there are no studies showing a significant difference in information content between the two types of waveforms.

Also, it is well known that nonrespiratory variables can profoundly influence the capnograph and thus the capnogram; they include, but are not limited to, type of anesthesia circuit, mode of ventilation, sampling site, sample flow rate, and fresh gas flow rate. [8–10]

A recent study of infrared carbon dioxide monitors showed that all could measure carbon dioxide at respiratory rates up to 60 breaths/min, and several up to 90 breaths/min.[4] Shared mass spectrometers, on the other hand, may have problems measuring rates much above 40 breaths/min[11]; the problems are many and may not be simply a function of response time. Mass spectrometers with a short sampling line can respond to respiratory rates of up to 330 breaths/minute.[12]

A recent report on techniques for measuring the time constants of mainstream and sidestream capnometers described a simple method for routine checking: quiet breathing followed by a 10-sec breath hold.[13] The expiratory flow after breathholding contains a step change in carbon dioxide. Recording the response on a fast recorder makes it possible to determine rise times. This same report described a study of the response of 10 instruments measured during ventilation at 20 to 100 breaths/min and at I:E ratios of 1:1 and 2:1. For breathing rates up to 60 breaths/min and an I:E ratio of 2:1, a 10 to 70% rise time should be at least 90 ms. For an I:E ratio of 1:1, a 10 to 70% rise time should be 160 ms. To measure 100 breaths/min, the 10 to 70% rise time should be less than 70 ms. Interestingly, 10 to 70% rise times were selected for measurement convenience and rise time is very close to the 0 to 63% or one time constant (1.098τ). These results confirm the frequently quoted objective that time constants of approximately 100 ms are needed for carbon dioxide monitoring.

The choice of sampling catheter material for shared mass spectrometers also profoundly influences response time.[12] For example, 30 M of nylon (0.86 mm ID) introduces a 10% error in end-tidal carbon dioxide at a breathing rate of 66 breaths/min, whereas a PVC catheter fails at 6 breaths/min, Teflon at 9 breaths/min, and polyethylene at 34 breaths/min. Such large differences can probably be explained by a gas absorption effect. The permeability of carbon dioxide (diffusion × solubility) with these materials is significantly greater than with nylon (Table 9.3).

Table 9.3 Carbon Dioxide Permeability of Materials Used for Sampling Catheters

Material	Permeability*
Nylon-6	10–12
Polyethylene (low-to-high density)	580–2700
Teflon†	110–1670
Polyvinyl chloride plasticizer	30–600

*cc-mil/100 square inch for 24 hours at 25°C.
†Fluoroplastics (ECTFE-GEP).

Unlike electrocardiography, no standards exist for guiding the clinician in response time requirements. However, one of the highest frequency repetitive signals on the capnogram has its origin in cardiac activity (cardiogenic oscillations, p. 27). The detection of that activity even at neonate heart rates of 200 beats/min can still be done at diminished amplitudes with a time constant of 100 ms.

Gas Diffusion

Both axial and radial diffusion of gas may contribute to waveform distortion at high breathing rates. Axial diffusion smears the upstroke of waveforms and they begin to merge together. This diffusion across the front and back boundaries of a gas sample has a larger effect on smaller volumes of gas and, thus, a greater effect at higher frequencies.

Radial diffusion of gas can be influenced by permeability of the catheter material. Carbon dioxide dissolves into the plastic and diffuses through the catheter wall to room air, where its partial pressure is low. This causes a gradient that promotes mass movement of gas out of the catheter. The longer the catheter, the greater the effect.[13]

Temperature

In infrared capnography the influence of temperature, an important consideration in measuring any gas, is relatively slight, only 0.3%/°C. This is because the temperature range of expired gas is small and its effect is controlled by the gas laws. Another issue related to temperature, however, is particularly important when end-tidal and blood gas values are compared, namely, the temperature of the patient, for which blood gas values must be corrected. The solubility of carbon dioxide in blood has a relatively high temperature coefficient (4.5%/°C).[14] For a patient at 35°C, the measured blood gas value at 37°C is 9.4% higher than true arterial carbon dioxide tension. When a mainstream capnograph measures carbon dioxide, it is 35°C, the temperature of the patient. The reading will be increased slightly (to 0.6%) because the temperature of the expired gas is 31°C, not the assumed temperature of 33°C for a patient at 37°C. However, the solubility effect causes end-tidal carbon dioxide to be 9.4% lower than the blood gas value measured at 37°C. Therefore, the apparent gradient is overestimated by 8.8% (3.5 mm Hg at an end-tidal carbon dioxide of 40 mm Hg). When gradients are measured, the blood gas value must always be corrected to the patient's temperature.

REFERENCES

1. Collier CR, Affeldt JE, Farr AF: Continuous rapid infrared CO_2 analysis. J Lab Clin Med 45:526–539, 1955

2. Luft K: Über eine neue Methode der registrierenden Gasanalyse mit Hilfe der Absorption ultraroter Strahlen ohne spektrale Zerlegung. Ztschr f Techn Phys 24:97, 1943

3. VanWagenen RA, Westenskow DR, Benner RG, et al: Dedicated monitoring of anesthetic and respiratory gases by Raman scattering. Int J Comput Monit 2:215–222, 1986

4. Anonymous: Evaluation: Carbon dioxide monitors. ECRI Health Dev 15:255–271, 1986

5. Severinghaus JW, Larson CP, Eger EI: Correction factors for infrared carbon dioxide pressure broadening by nitrogen, nitrous oxide and cyclopropane. Anesthesiology 22:429–432, 1961

6. Ammann ECB, Galvin RD: Problems associated with the determination of carbon dioxide by infrared absorption. J Appl Physiol 25:333–335, 1968

7. Solomon RJ: A reliable, accurate CO_2 analyzer for medical use. Hewlett-Packard J 32:3–21, 1981

8. Gravenstein N, Lampotang S, Beneken JEW: Factors influencing capnography in the Bain circuit. J Clin Monit 1:6–10, 1985

9. Schieber RA, Namnoum A, Sugden A, Saville AL, Orr RA: Accuracy of expiratory carbon dioxide measurements using the coaxial and circle breathing circuits in small subjects. J Clin Monit 1:149–155, 1985

10. Sasse FJ: Can we trust end-tidal carbon dioxide measurements in infants. J Clin Monit 1:147–148, 1985

11. Meny RG, Bhat AM, Aranas E: Mass spectrometer monitoring of expired carbon dioxide in critically ill neonates. Crit Care Med 13:1064–1066, 1985

12. Scamman FL, Fishbaugh JK: Frequency response of long mass-spectrometer sampling catheters. Anesthesiology 65:422–425, 1986

13. Brunner JX, Westenskow DR: How carbon dioxide rise time affects the accuracy of carbon dioxide measurements. J Clin Monit 4:134, 1988

14. Severinghaus JW, Stafford M, Bradley AF: $tcPCO_2$ electrode design, calibration and temperature gradient problems. Acta Anaesthesiol Scand [Suppl] 68:118–122, 1978

Chapter 10

Capnometry Based on Spectral Techniques: Infrared and Raman

The electromagnetic spectrum can be described by wavelength (λ), wave number ($1/\lambda$), and frequency ($\nu = c/\lambda$, where c is the velocity of light). Infrared spectroscopists use wave number because it is proportional to energy:

$$E = h\nu = h\frac{c}{\lambda}$$

where h is Planck's constant. This relationship is a reminder that higher energy quanta have higher frequencies, higher wave numbers, and shorter wavelengths. Some of these frequencies have enough energy to ionize molecules (roentgen and ultraviolet), some are absorbed and cause chemical reactions (ultraviolet and visible), and some influence the vibration and rotation of molecules (infrared). The infrared spectrum begins just beyond the red part of the visible spectrum (0.4 to 0.8 μ) and extends to approximately 40 μ.

INFRARED

The infrared part of the spectrum has some distinct advantages for medical monitoring. Infrared is safe because it causes no permanent changes in the molecule. The absorption of infrared energy increases molecular rotation and vibration, which increases temperature, but only modestly. Therefore, infrared can be used on-line if necessary to measure respiratory gases. Blackbody radiators heated to moderate temperatures can be used to radiate infrared energy, which can be detected by a host of solid state devices. Materials that can transmit infrared are readily available for windows and filters. In other words, infrared instruments are simple and relatively inexpensive.

This spectral region is particularly appropriate for measuring carbon dioxide because it has a strong absorption band in the near infrared (4.26 μ), which lies between two strong bands for water vapor (Figure 10.1) and yet is distinct enough from the main bands of most other potentially interfering agents (halothane, 13.95μ; enflurane, 12.2; isoflurane, 8.55, 11.06, and 12.95) to minimize interference; all these have a common band at 3.3; the band for nitrous oxide, however, is close enough to cause a problem. Carbon monoxide concentrations generally are very low. Even when the concentration of car-boxyhemoglobin is high, the concentration of carbon monoxide is in the parts per million range. Oxygen and nitrogen do not have infrared absorption bands but, nevertheless, can influence absorption through a pressure or line broad-ening effect.

Carbon Dioxide and Infrared Absorption

In order to absorb infrared radiation, a molecule must be both asymmetric and polyatomic. Atoms or molecules such as helium, argon, hydrogen, oxygen, and nitrogen do not satisfy these requirements and therefore do not absorb;

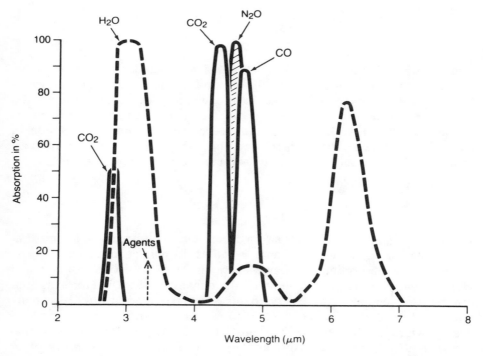

FIGURE 10.1   *Absorption bands for some common gases in the near infrared, for band location only, as measurement conditions vary. Agents refer to halothane, enflurane, and isoflurane. (From Craver CD: A Special Collection of Infrared Spectra from The Coblentz Society, Inc. Kirkwood, MO, The Coblentz Society, 1980.)*

carbon dioxide, nitrous oxide, and water do. Molecular asymmetry does not simply mean that different atoms exist in the same molecule. It also means that allowed infrared vibrations will cause centers of electrical charge to be displaced; in other words, an allowed vibration will alter the molecule's dipole moment. Carbon dioxide is a good example of the principles involved because it has both symmetric and asymmetric vibrations. The frequency with which these vibrations occur depends on the masses of the atoms as well as the strength of the bond holding the atoms together. These vibrations occur at frequencies on the order of 10^{13}/sec. This corresponds to frequencies found within the infrared part of the spectrum. Absorption of infrared energy simply increases the amplitude of the vibration but does not change its frequency. Because a linear molecule with n atoms has $3n - 5$ fundamental vibrations, carbon dioxide ($[3 \cdot 3] - 5$) must have four fundamental vibrational modes

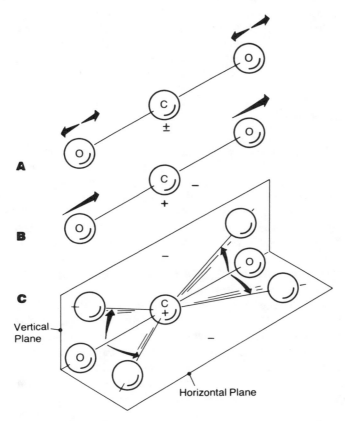

FIGURE 10.2 *Vibrational frequencies for carbon dioxide. (A) Symmetric vibration with no displacement of electric charge and therefore infrared inactive. (B) Asymmetric vibration that displaces electric charge and is infrared active (4.26 μ). (C) Bending vibration that displaces electric charge and is infrared active (15 μ).*

(Figure 10.2). The first is a symmetric stretch vibration, which does not change the dipole moment of the molecule and is therefore not infrared-active. The second is an asymmetric stretch vibration and is infrared-active. During the vibration the center of negative charge is displaced from the center of positive charge. This wave band at 2349 cm^{-1} (4.26 μ) is used in most monitors.

Further, there are two bending modes, which can occur in the horizontal or the vertical plane (Figure 10.2C). Again, the centers of negative charge move in the respective planes as the bending action occurs. In a vibrational sense, the bending modes are infrared active and degenerate; that is they have the same wave number, namely, 667 cm^{-1} (14.99 μ).

In summary, for carbon dioxide two infrared-active fundamental vibrations are predicted and two are found: one (asymmetric mode) at 2349 cm^{-1} (4.26 μ) and the other (bending mode) at 667 cm^{-1} (14.99 μ). There is another wave band at 3846 cm^{-1} (2.6 μ), which is an overtone band and is a combination of the fundamental vibrational frequencies. It is fortunate that the high-intensity wave band for carbon dioxide at 4.26 μ lies between the two very intense bands for water. With carefully characterized, narrow-band pass optical filters, carbon dioxide can be measured with little interference either from water vapor or from the neighboring band for nitrous oxide.

Pressure Broadening

As we have seen, infrared absorption is a measure of vibrational frequencies of atoms within a molecule. These vibrations are a function of factors both internal and external to the molecule. Internally, frequency depends mostly on the strength of the bond between atoms and their relative masses. Externally, spatial arrangement of atoms, intermolecular forces, and collisions between molecules influence the frequency of vibrations. All these factors may alter the shape of the absorption bands. As we have also seen, vibration determines band location. Associated with the principal bands are a number of other bands that are related to the rotation of a molecule. These bands are usually small and are sometimes called rotational bands or side bands. Side bands become more prominent as the frequency of collisions, or the level of pressure, increases. Pressure, or collision, broadening is the reason these gases do not follow Beer's law (as first observed by Ångstrom in 1890). The ability of a diluent gas to absorb energy from an excited carbon dioxide molecule also affects pressure broadening. Consequently, a calibration curve depends not only on total pressure but also on the constituents of the gas mixture as well. Change the constituents, and the curve changes.

Over the years a number of conclusions about the influence of pressure broadening on carbon dioxide absorption have been reached.

1. The pressure broadening influence on carbon dioxide is in the following order: helium, argon < oxygen, < nitrogen, < nitrous oxide < H_2.[1,2] Absorp-

tion can be enhanced most for H_2 and least for the monatomic gases, helium and argon.

2. The absolute magnitude of pressure broadening depends on the design of the measuring instrument[1] and is controlled by source, filter, and detector.

3. The relative influence of any gas on a specific instrument will be about the same[1]; therefore, if the influence of a specific gas is known, the influence of others can be estimated from reported data (Table 10.1).[2] For example, if the influence of oxygen on an instrument is found to be 3% (*i.e.*, K = 1.03), then the influence of helium would be expected to be 5.5% (K = 1.055) when N_2 is the reference gas.

4. Pressure broadening is independent of the concentration of carbon dioxide up to 10% for single diluent gases.

5. For mixtures of gases, the effect on each gas is complex, *i.e.*, not linear.[3,4]

Pressure broadening then must be considered when gases other than the calibrating gas are to be measured.

INSTRUMENTATION

Having considered some of the characteristics of infrared measurements, a review of the types of measuring systems is appropriate. All infrared instruments consist basically of a radiation source, a cell through which samples of gas flow, and a detector that transmits a signal related to the intensity of the radiation that is detected. The quantitative aspects of photometric measurement are stated by the Beer-Lambert law:

$$A = \log (I_o/I) = \epsilon lc$$

Under carefully controlled conditions at a select absorption band, the absorbance of a sample (A) is proportional both to the concentration of sample (c) and the depth of the absorbing layer (l). The molar extinction coefficient (ϵ)

Table 10.1 Pressure Broadening Correction Factors (K) for Various Gases

Diluent Gas	K
Helium or argon	1.11
Oxygen	1.06
Nitrogen	1.00
Hydrogen	0.87

Multiplying the measurement in various diluent gases by K corrects to a calibration curve where the diluent gas is nitrogen; this is valid only with a Beckman IR215 analyzer.

is a wavelength-dependent constant characterizing the sample. I_o is the intensity of radiation with no sample in the beam and I intensity with a sample. For solutions, absorbances are additive. Absorbance then is also minus the log of the transmittance ($A = -\log T$), which denotes that the relationship between concentration and transmittance is nonlinear. Transmittance approaches zero as concentration approaches infinity. However, there is a part of the range that is close to linear (Figure 10.3).

In the infrared region gases do not follow the Beer-Lambert law because of a pressure broadening effect. Both total pressure and diluent gases influence the side bands and thus the amount of radiation absorbed. However, under controlled conditions calibration curves can be constructed, the influence of perturbations studied, and quantitations made.

Nondispersive Infrared Capnometers

Most continuous monitors of carbon dioxide are of the nondispersive infrared (NDIR) type; there is no provision for dispersing the radiation into its com-

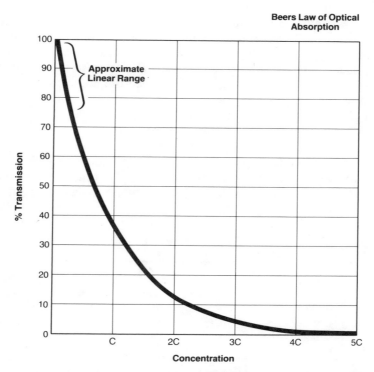

FIGURE 10.3   *Beer's law of optical absorption predicts an exponential decrease in transmission with increasing concentration. Over some small range, the relationship is almost linear.*

ponent wavelengths. The technique, developed during World War II by Luft in Germany and Pfund and Gemmill in the United States,[5,6] was first used in the rubber industry and for environmental monitoring in submarines. By the early 1950s these instruments were adapted for medical purposes.

Single-Beam

The earliest NDIR instruments were characterized by their use of broad-band energy from a blackbody source; no attempt was made at wavelength selection (Figure 10.4). Incoherent radiation—incoherent because it contains many wavelengths—from an infrared source is transmitted through a sample cell to an infrared-sensitive detector. When an infrared absorber (for example, carbon dioxide) appears in the sample cell, the intensity of radiation reaching the broadband detector decreases, which in turn diminishes the signal. This type of system is not specific but, because of the high intensity light, is stable. This instrument could be reasonably useful in a well-defined process; for example, an NDIR single-beam capnometer could readily be used to control a single absorbing constituent in a process involving no other infrared absorbers. Because they are simpler, less costly, and more rugged than dispersive instruments, NDIR instruments are preferred for industrial monitoring. These same advantages are also important for medical monitoring.

Double-Beam Positive-Filter

Both stability and specificity are improved by adding a second beam and a selective detector (Figure 10.5). These improvements are based on two innovations in design. First, specificity is improved because the detector responds only to radiation specifically influenced by carbon dioxide. This is done by filling the detector with carbon dioxide; thus, only the radiation that comes through the reference or sample cell and is absorbed by the carbon dioxide in the detector is measured. Carbon dioxide in the sample cell decreases the radiation and the signal. The capnometer transduces the signal by measuring a change in capacitance that results from the displacement of a thin diaphragm either optically or by considering the diaphragm as one plate of a parallel plate capacitor.[5] The diaphragm is displaced by an increase in pressure caused by heating, and the heat results from the absorption of infrared radiation by the

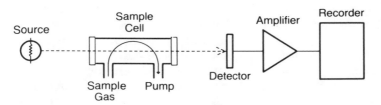

FIGURE 10.4 *Nondispersive, infrared, single-beam capnometer. The source and detector are broad-band and nonselective. This design would work if carbon dioxide were the only absorber in the sample gas.*

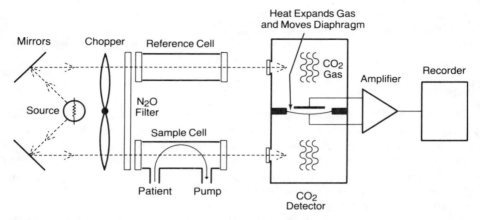

FIGURE 10.5   *Nondispersive, infrared, double-beam capnometer. The addition of a reference cell and selective detector provides source monitoring and sensitivity to a specific gas (i.e., carbon dioxide). Overlapping absorption from nitrous oxide can be removed by adding a filter to absorb the radiation in the nitrous oxide absorption band.*

carbon dioxide. The second improvement, greater overall stability, results from a reference beam that monitors the source output; the reference cell contains a nonabsorbing gas, *e.g.*, nitrogen. A specially designed chopper periodically permits measurement of reference signal, sample signal, and dark signal.

This kind of detector, known as the Luft cell, can be traced to the "photoacoustic effect" first observed by Alexander Graham Bell in 1880.[7] He placed test gases (cigar smoke) in a test tube, irradiated it with a chopped beam of light and, via a rubber tube connected to the test tube, detected audible signal. The photoacoustic effect is the sound emitted when an enclosed sample of gas absorbs light chopped in the audible range (20 Hz to 20 kHz). This observation led to the development of photoacoustic spectroscopy, which is used today in the design of highly sensitive environmental monitors. In place of the ear, microphones have been developed that convert chopped radiation into an alternating voltage. Because capacitance is inversely proportional to the distance between the plates (as in the parallel plate capacitor in the Luft cell), and voltage is inversely proportional to capacitance, then the AC voltage can be used to replicate pressure and to measure concentration. Whether it is the Luft cell or photoacoustics, the underlying mechanism is the same—changes in pressure resulting from the absorption of infrared energy.

Another way of designing a carbon dioxide detector is to use a solid-state sensor that has broad spectral sensitivity and an optical filter that transmits radiation in the 4.26-μ region. These filters can be made with bandwidths that are quite narrow, 5% of the peak wavelength at 50% transmission. The best

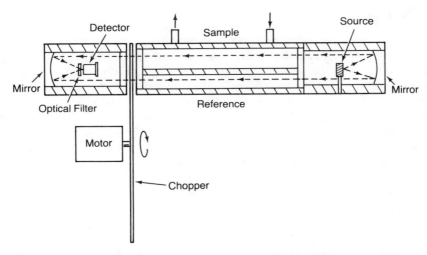

FIGURE 10.6 *An NDIR optical bench showing a reference cell and a selective solid state detector. Broad-band radiation from the source is collimated by the mirror and passes through both reference and sample cell. The chopper modulates the light beam and makes possible the monitoring of sample, reference, and dark signals, from which the partial pressure of carbon dioxide can be determined.*

detector for carbon dioxide is lead selenide because of its broad spectral response in the near infrared. It is sometimes thermoelectrically cooled to improve signal to noise.

Double-beam capnometers* (Figure 10.6) produce conventional signals; that is, the signal increases as the concentration of carbon dioxide increases. Signal is defined as the difference between the reference beam signal and the sample beam signal. This type of system is more completely described as an NDIR system of the positive filter type. Some sidestream capnometers are of this design.

Other sidestream designs use a single beam with a rotating filter wheel.** This has the advantage of combining the signal modulation produced by the chopper with multi-gas monitoring, as well as source and sample cell monitoring with a reference cell. Appropriate optical filters are mounted in the wheel along with a reference cell. Each revolution provides the necessary optical information to calculate gas concentrations.

* Sensors, Incorporated
  6812 South Street Road
  Saline, MI 48176
**Andros Analyzers
  2332 Fourth Street
  Berkeley, CA 94710

Double-Beam Negative-Filter

With this capnometric implementation (Figure 10.7),[6] the sample gas is measured in series with a cell that contains no carbon dioxide (*e.g.*, nitrogen) and in series with a cell that contains a high concentration of carbon dioxide. The high concentration of carbon dioxide absorbs most of the radiation in the carbon dioxide band. Therefore, the sample carbon dioxide makes little difference in signal (V_R); however, the sample carbon dioxide in series with the nitrogen cell does produce a significant signal (V_S). This is an unconventional approach because the difference between the two signals ($V_S - V_R$) is greatest when there is no carbon dioxide in the sample. Increasing concentrations decrease this V_S and the difference; signal to noise also decreases. Usually noise is a concern when concentration approaches zero. However, design parameters can be selected such that the physiological range can be measured with an acceptable signal to noise ratio. In some implementations, the ratio V_R/V_S can be measured. This has the advantage of increasing as concentration increases. Again, a chopper makes it possible for both beams to be served by a single source and detector.

With some rearrangement of the parts, it is possible to see how this principle might be applied to mainstream capnometers (Figure 10.8). The sample chamber is located in the breathing circuit as close to the mouth or endotracheal tube as possible. The infrared beam passes through the sample chamber and before reaching the detector must pass through the filter wheel. This is possible only during two periods of each revolution. One is when the carbon dioxide-containing cell is in the beam and the other is when the nitrogen or blank cell is in the beam; thus, two signals are generated. The ratio of the two signals (V_R/V_S) is used to track the concentration of carbon dioxide in the sample chamber. The rotation of the filter wheel modulates the infrared beam and

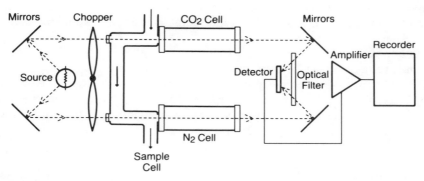

FIGURE 10.7 *An NDIR negative-filter, double-beam capnometer. The addition of sample carbon dioxide to the carbon dioxide reference cell causes only a small change in signal compared to sample cell carbon dioxide added to the nitrogen cell. The difference between the nitrogen cell signal and the carbon dioxide cell signal decreases as the concentration of carbon dioxide in the sample gas increases.*

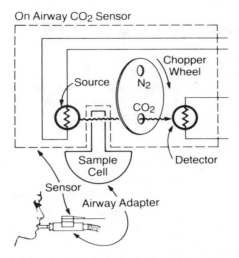

On Airway CO₂ Sensor

FIGURE 10.8 *An NDIR negative-filter, single-beam capnometer. The carbon dioxide cell and nitrogen cell are mounted in a chopper wheel that rotates in front of the sample cell. This provides continuous monitoring of sample cell condition, as well as source.*

thus performs the same function as the chopper, allowing dark as well as reference cell measurements; an additional advantage is that the sample cell can be monitored.

The Chopper

In many capnometric implementations a chopper is used; this technique not only makes possible the use of a common source and detector in the double-beam types but has the added advantage of producing an alternating signal, one from the sample beam and one from the reference beam. The information contained in the difference between these two signals is usually too small to drive display devices and recorders; consequently, the signals are amplified by a differential amplifier that increases the difference between two signals. Also, the amplifier is designed not to react to signals that are the same; for example, when there is no carbon dioxide in the sample cell, reference and sample signals should be the same. Another consideration is that the carbon dioxide-containing signal may be only a small part of the total signal. If it is not chopped, drift could obscure information. Checking the reference cell by frequently chopping the signal can prevent this problem. A third benefit is a reduction in interference that would affect both reference and sample cell signals. For example, 60-Hz signals from a power line picked up either in cables or from stray light would be rejected. The ability of the circuit design to reject such unwanted signals is referred to as common mode rejection ratio (CMRR), a specification often used for electrocardiographs.

Calibration

NDIR, On-Airway

For calibration, measurements are made when carbon dioxide in the sample chamber is zero and when it is at some midscale value. This is done in two ways: either with a calibrating gas flowing through the airway or with stable calibrating cells containing the appropriate gases, which can be substituted for the sample chamber.[3]

In one mainstream device[8] the airway sample chamber serves as the reference cell during inhalation (Figure 10.9). Just as the reference cell in sidestream NDIR instruments makes it possible to compensate for such problems as instabilities in source and detector, clouded windows, and amplifier drift, so this sample cell can serve the same purpose. Notice that the chopper simply modulates this light beam and is not responsible for sample switching. This is done by the breathing cycle. When inspiratory gas enters the sample chamber, the low value is assumed to be zero as would be the case with a conventional double-beam instrument with a true zero reference cell.

This strategy, however, will work only when there is no carbon dioxide in the inspiratory gas as is true for the Siemens and many other ventilators. Such capnometric devices cannot detect rebreathing. In the operating room saturated

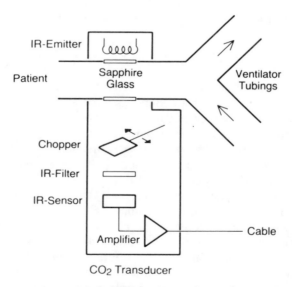

FIGURE 10.9   *A mainstream NDIR positive-filter capnometer. This is a double-beam implementation that depends on the respiratory cycle. The reference beam is the patient gas during inhalation, which normally contains no carbon dioxide. (Reproduced with permission from Olsson SG, Fletcher R, Jonson B, et al: Clinical studies of gas exchange during ventilatory support—a method using Siemens–Elema CO$_2$ analyzer. Br J Anaesth 52:491–499, 1980.)*

carbon dioxide absorbers, failed expiratory valves, and increased dead space also will not be detected. However, these capnometers respond very quickly, and when the capnographic data are integrated with flow waveforms, carbon dioxide production can be measured accurately.

Dispersive Techniques

Infrared radiation can be dispersed into its component wavelengths with a prism or a grating. A means for scanning the spectrum and measuring absorption is also provided. This type of instrument is used primarily for research and in industrial laboratories. At present, dispersive infrared instruments are not used in medical monitoring.

RAMAN SCATTERING

Just as absorption of infrared energy can increase rotational and vibrational activity of molecules, so can absorption of visible or ultraviolet radiation. Predicted by Smekal in 1923 and confirmed by Raman and Krishnan in 1928, the phenomenon is called Raman scattering. Radiation scattering can occur in several ways. The clear manifestation of a beam of light by means of airborne dust is an example of scattering by particles that are large relative to the wavelength of light (Tyndall effect). When the scattered particles are small (molecules), a different kind of scattering occurs. It is an absorption–re-emission phenomenon, in which there is no change in wavelength, and occurs instantaneously, within 10^{-12} sec (Rayleigh). Although wavelength does not change, shorter wavelengths are more stimulating. This explains why the sky appears blue; the shorter blue wavelengths in sunlight are preferentially scattered, which increases the intensity of that wavelength as it reaches earth.

Another kind of absorption–re-emission scattering can cause a wavelength change. This indicates that radiation in the visible part of the spectrum is only partially absorbed, which increases the amplitude of a molecular vibration. The remaining energy is re-emitted at a longer, or slightly shifted, wavelength (lower frequency) as is required by conservation of energy. Recall that rotational and vibrational energy levels normally are activated by the absorption of infrared radiation.

This wavelength shifting with partial absorption was surprising because it violated a well-established belief concerning absorption spectroscopy: the fundamental rule that the absorption of radiant energy occurs only for those photons that have energy corresponding precisely to an allowable transition within atoms or molecules. Allowable transitions define the absorption spectra, wavelengths that are shorter normally being no more effective than wavelengths that are longer in causing these transitions. An exception is Raman scattering,[9] where wavelengths in the visible spectrum or ultraviolet range can be partially absorbed, which increases rotational and vibrational activity. The probability of this kind of absorption is very low and, consequently, the intensity of the scattered radiation is low.

Raman scattering is similar to fluorescence, where the wavelength of fluoresced light is longer than that of the exciting light. Because Stokes has been identified with this observation, the Raman line with a wavelength longer than the incident or exciting line is called a Stokes' line. The other relationship is also possible: the scattered wavelength can be shorter than the incident, and that is called an anti-Stokes' line (Figure 10.10). This kind of transition does not occur very often because at room temperature most gas molecules are in their ground state (ν_0) and only a few are in an excited state (ν_1). The change in wavelength, or frequency shift, depends on the vibrational and rotational

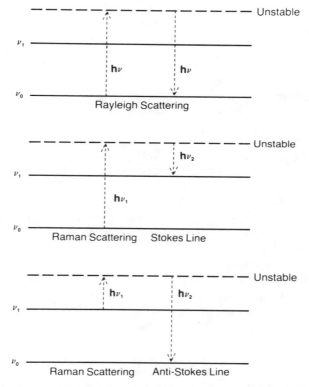

FIGURE 10.10 *Energy level diagrams showing molecular scattering. Rayleigh scattering: instantaneous re-emission of an absorbed photon ν with no change in wavelength. Raman scattering Stokes' line: instantaneous re-emission of a photon with a lower frequency (longer wavelength) than the absorbed photon. Raman scattering, anti-Stokes' line: instantaneous re-emission of a photon with a higher frequency (shorter wavelength) than the absorbed photon. All transitions are from a ground state (ν_0) or from a stable vibrational level (ν_1) to an unstable level (---).*

levels of the scattering molecule and are unique for each molecule; therefore, the shift can be used for identification purposes. In addition, the intensity of the Raman line relates to concentration; thus, quantitation is also possible.

Over the years Raman scattering has been used to study molecular structure, the information complementing that gained from infrared. It has been complementary because the selection rules governing allowable transitions among energy level for infrared are not the same as they are for Raman. For example, oxygen and nitrogen, which do not have absorption bands in the infrared, are Raman-active. This is precisely because the symmetric vibrations that are excluded from infrared are the basis for Raman activity. Therefore, all physiologic gases as well as all anesthetic gases are measurable; monatomic gases, which do not have a vibrational structure, are not.

By definition, both the Raman and Rayleigh transitions produce scattered light, and so, must be measured off the path of incident light, usually at right angles. Again, the intensity is usually very low. A rule of thumb is that only 0.1% of the incident light is scattered. Of that, only 0.1% experiences a Raman shift; therefore, about 1 in a million photons are scattered with a change in wavelength. Early investigators used mercury vapor lamps and long exposures of fast photographic emulsions. These have given way to high-intensity, forced air cooled argon lasers and sensitive photomultiplier tubes.

For multiple gas analysis, resolution is a potential problem (Table 10.2).[10] For the gases used or monitored during anesthesia, the spectral range is a little less than 100 nm. The agents are particularly close together in a range of 7.2 nm. Also, some interference would be expected between nitrogen and nitrous oxide. The usual approach of separating these bands by using monochromators is too expensive and unwieldy for an operating room monitor. Using narrow band-pass filters with a frequency width at half-maximum (FWHM) of 1 nm has enough resolving power to make the system workable, although overlap is

Table 10.2 Raman Frequency Shifts Applied to Radiation from an Argon Laser Wave No. 20,492 cm^{-1} (488 nm)

Gas	Frequency Shift Wave No. (cm^{-1})	Wave Length (nm)
Halothane	717	505.7
Enflurane	817	508.3
Isoflurane	995	512.9
Carbon dioxide	1285	520.6
Nitrous oxide	1285	520.6
Carbon dioxide	1388	523.4
Oxygen	1555	528.1
Nitrous oxide	2224	547.4
Nitrogen	2331	550.6
Water	3650	593.8

not eliminated. The use of microprocessors and empirically determined algorithms has provided impressive results in bench testing of a prototype instrument (Figure 10.11).[10]

The use of Raman scattering is new to medical gas monitoring. The technique has been bench tested,[11] and further refinements of design have yielded a prototype instrument.[10] All these data look encouraging: accuracy, rise time, and stability specifications meet clinical needs. In the present design carbon dioxide is measured continuously by a separate photomultiplier tube. A second photomultiplier tube disposed at a right angle on the other side of the sample cell measures oxygen, nitrogen, nitrous oxide, and anesthetic agents. These measurements are discontinuous. Design changes to provide continuous monitoring for eight gases and improvements in response time by means of a reduction in sample cell volume are reported to be in process.

Interference from other gases, *e.g.*, bronchodilators, has not been investigated as yet. Although it is probable that exposure to high-energy radiation at 488 nm does not significantly affect any of the gases, this must be checked carefully because there may be some low-level photochemical activity. This question may be moot because there is an increasing reluctance to recycle gases through the anesthesia circuit because of the possibility of cross-contamination.

Raman is new and exciting. It holds the promise of a dedicated multigas

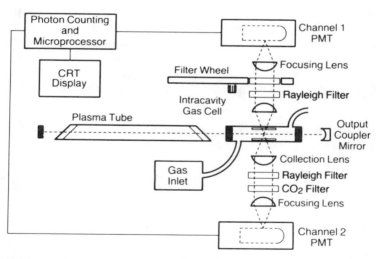

FIGURE 10.11   *Raman instrumentation. The argon laser (plasma tube) irradiates the sample, which is aspirated through the gas cell. The Rayleigh filters are used to block the scattered but unshifted laser wavelength. Appropriate narrow band filters mounted in the filter wheel monitor six gases in Channel 1. Carbon dioxide is monitored continuously in Channel 2. High sensitivity photomultiplier tubes (PMT) are used for detection. (Reproduced with permission from VanWegenen RA, Westenskow DR, Benner RE, et al: Dedicated monitoring of anesthetic and respiratory gases by Raman scattering. J Clin Monit 2:215–222, 1986.)*

monitor for operating room and bedside use, which is affordable, simpler than mass spectrometry, and more comprehensive than infrared.

REFERENCES

1. Severinghaus JW, Larson CP, Eger EI: Correction factors for infrared carbon dioxide pressure broadening by N_2, N_2O and cyclopropane. Anesthesiology 22:429–432, 1961
2. Ammann ECB, Galvin RD: Problems associated with the determination of carbon dioxide by infrared absorption. J Appl Physiol 25:333–335, 1968
3. Solomon RJ: A reliable, accurate CO_2 analyzer for medical use. Hewlett Packard J 32:3–21, 1981
4. Elam JO, Brown ES, Ten Pas RH: Carbon dioxide hemostasis during anesthesia; I. Instrumentation. Anesthesiology 16:876–885, 1955
5. Luft K: Über eine neue Methode der registrierenden Gasanalyse mit Hilfe der Absorption ultraroter Strahlen ohne spektrale Zerlegung. Ztschr f Techn Phys 24:97, 1943
6. Pfund AH, Gemmill CL: An infrared absorption method for the quantitative analysis of respiratory and other gases. Bull Johns Hopkins Hosp 67:61–65, 1940
7. Anonymous: Photoacoustics in Gas Detection. Supplied by Bruel and Kjaer, 2850, Naerum, Denmark
8. Olsson SG, Fletcher R, Jonson B, et al: Clinical studies of gas exchange during ventilatory support—a method using the Siemens–Elema CO_2 analyzer. Br J Anaesth 52:491–499, 1980
9. Bauman RP: Absorption Spectroscopy. New York, Wiley, 1962
10. VanWagenen RA, Westenskow DR, Benner RE, et al: Dedicated monitoring of anesthetic and respiratory gases by Raman scattering. J Clin Monit 2:215–222, 1986
11. VanWagenen R, Westenskow DR, Benner R: Respiratory gas analysis by Raman scattering. Anesthesiology 63:A163, 1985

Chapter 11

Capnometry Based on Molecular Weight: Mass Spectrometry

HISTORICAL DEVELOPMENT OF THE SPECTROMETER

As with many technologic developments now being applied routinely in clinical practice, mass spectrometry has its origins in the early part of this century. The idea of separating charged particles (ions) by their mass was first proposed and practically applied by J.J. Thompson and F.W. Aston, who used the technique in isotope research.[1] The technical evolution of that idea from a laboratory tool useful in many fields of research to a practical clinical instrument required 50 years of experience, the prodding and support of the National Aeronautics and Space Administration (NASA), and the vision of early medical users who recognized its potential.

Researchers through the 1950s and 1960s were quick to take advantage of the mass spectrometer to measure several gases simultaneously.[2] It was used to clarify and explore some basic questions in respiratory physiology and to improve pulmonary function testing. These applications made mass spectrometric principles familiar to physicians, but its more general use as a clinical monitor rested upon developments at NASA. NASA support of mass spectrometry as the appropriate technique for monitoring respiratory gases, planetary atmospheres, and closed environments in outer space resulted in the development of small, rugged, and reliable instruments. These systems were more accepted for monitoring in the intensive care unit, at least initially, because the gases to be monitored were relatively simple. In the operating room detecting nitrous oxide and carbon dioxide is problematic because both gases have approximately the same mass. A mass spectrometer with the resolving power to separate them would be too expensive. Measuring other anesthetic agents was also a problem at first because the mass range was generally less than 150 amu. By the early 1980s these sampling and detection problems were resolved and reliability was improved; in 1981 mass spectrometry became established as a cost-effective and reliable monitor for operating room use.[3]

127

PRINCIPLES OF MASS SPECTROMETRY

Two types of mass spectrometers have become important medically: the magnetic sector with fixed detectors and the quadrupole. Each has been used either as a dedicated instrument providing continuous monitoring of single patients or as a shared instrument (multiplexed) providing discontinuous monitoring of several patients in sequence.

Magnetic Sector—Fixed Detector

Sample gas is aspirated into a vacuum chamber and, there, is ionized by an electron beam (Figure 11.1). The charged fragments are accelerated by an electric field into a dispersion chamber where they are separated according to mass by a magnetic field. In mathematical terms, a particle of mass m with charge e accelerated through a voltage V acquires a kinetic energy eV

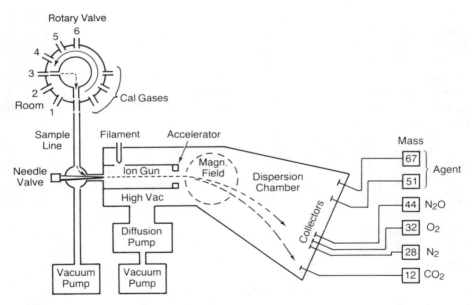

FIGURE 11.1 *Shared mass spectrometer—magnetic sector with fixed detectors. Patient gases and calibration gases are sequentially sampled by means of the rotary valve. A low flow into the mass spectrometer is controlled by a needle valve or molecular leak. Here the gas molecules are charged and fragmented by an electron beam, accelerated in an electric field, and dispersed in a magnetic field. Discrete detectors in the focal plane (collectors) measure the component gases. Carbon dioxide is measured as C^+, and nitrous oxide as N_2O^+. Anesthetic agents are identified by the ratio of fragments with masses 67/51.*

$$eV = \frac{1}{2} mv^2$$

where v is the velocity of the ion after acceleration. In the dispersion chamber a magnetic field of strength B is imposed at right angles to the direction of motion, which produces a deflecting force (evB) on the ions, which is normal to their direction of motion. This causes them to move in a circular path. The deflection force, then, is equal to centrifugal force

$$evB = \frac{mv^2}{r}$$

where r is the radius of the circular path. Eliminating v between the first two equations

$$r = \left(\frac{2mV}{eB^2}\right)1/2$$

This tells us that, if the accelerating voltage V and magnetic field strength B are held constant, the radius of the curved path depends only on the charge and the mass, or the m/e ratio. Particles (ions) with different m/e will have different radii. Lighter particles will move off-axis more quickly than heavier ones and, thus, separation is achieved. Detectors that measure the ion current from a particular mass fragment are placed at specific locations in the focal plane of the mass spectrometer.

FLOW REGIONS

To ensure accurate measurements, close attention should be paid to the gas flow characteristics in each of the three flow regions in a mass spectrometer: the molecular flow region in the dispersion chamber, the viscous flow region in the sampling lines, and the transitional region at the sampling valve.

Molecular Flow Region

Ion currents at the detector plates must be predictably related to the fractional composition of the gas at the sampling site; therefore, the sample cannot be altered in its composition as it makes its journey through the system. This means that the environment in the dispersion chamber becomes most important. Ideally, an ion travels from source to detector without colliding with any other molecule or ion. This happens at gas pressures less than 10^{-5} mm Hg where the mean free path (MFP), or distances traveled between collisions, is long compared with the trajectory of the ion or dimensions of the chamber. This flow region is known as the molecular flow region. Although MFP is different for each type of gas because the sizes of the molecules differ, an idea of its magnitude can be gleaned from an approximation of MFP for air[4]:

$$MFP = \frac{5}{\text{pressures in microns}}$$

For example, at a pressure of 1 μ (1 $\times$ 10^{-3} mm Hg), the MFP is 5 cm, or approximately 2 inches.

Viscous Flow Region

Pressures in the sample line are much higher than in the dispersion chamber; also, the MFP is much shorter and collisions occur more frequently. Intermolecular forces and viscosity play an important role in defining flow characteristics within the sampling system. For example, in a tube with a radius a (cm), a length L (cm), and a pressure drop $(P_1 - P_2)$ (dynes/cm^2), the flow Q (molecules/sec) of a gas with a viscosity of η (poise) is described by the following relationship (Poiseuille's equation):

$$Q = \frac{a^4(P_1\text{-}P_2)^2}{16 \; L\eta kT}$$

where k is the Boltzman constant (1.38 $\times$ 10^{-16} ERG/$^\circ$K per molecule) and T is the absolute temperature ($^\circ$K). There is a strong dependence of flow on the size of the tube. Doubling the radius increases flow 16 times.

There is a transitional region between viscous and molecular flow where container dimensions are 2 to 25 times the value of MFP. The pressure drop of a gas moving from a region of viscous to a region of molecular flow will be influenced by both the viscosity of the gas and its molecular weight.[2] The molecular weight dependence would alter the distribution of gases in the dispersion chamber, but probably could be accounted for in the processing. All these flow regions are represented in a mass spectrometer, and must be integrated to insure that a measuring system can maintain sample integrity and can provide accurate information on gas composition.

PRESSURE GRADIENTS/SAMPLE FLOW

The sample in the dispersion chamber where the pressure is 10^{-6} to 10^{-7} mm Hg comes from the ionization chamber where pressure is on the order of 10^{-5} mm Hg. In this pressure region,

$$P_D = K_1 P_I$$

where P_D is dispersion chamber pressure, K_1 is a proportionality constant, and P_I is ionization chamber pressure.

Sample gas enters the ionization chamber through what is commonly referred to as a "molecular leak." The flow characteristics of this leak are very important in maintaining an accurate relationship between the ion currents and the composition of the gas. In other words, the flow across the leak should be molecular such that

$$P_I = K_2 P_S$$

where P_I is the partial pressure in the ionization chamber, K_2 is a proportionality constant, and P_S is the partial pressure in the sample chamber. Here conflicting requirements come into play. In order to ensure molecular flow, the pressure in the sample chamber should be less than 0.1 mm Hg. For a pressure that low, the "viscous balancing" of the sampling system is disturbed. This problem relates to the way the sample is transported. First a separate pump is required that does not have to meet the technical requirements of an ion or oil diffusion pump because very low pressures are not necessary. The sampling pump must aspirate a small sample of gas from the patient (flow rate, 1 to 4 ml/sec) through a long capillary (100-foot) to a sample chamber where the molecular leak provides an escape path for a small fraction of the flow (10^{-4} ml/sec). The pump then discharges the gas sample to the atmosphere or to the hospital scavenging system.

The pressure drop across the sampling system is the problem, *i.e.*, from atmospheric pressure at the sampling site to the pressure at the sample pump (Figure 11.2). If flow throughout is viscous, then an increase in viscosity will decrease flow but will not affect fractional pressures along the capillary tube. The fractional pressure in the sample chamber, for example, bears a fixed relationship to atmospheric pressure and is independent of viscosity. Flow decreases when viscosity increases, but the pressure profile is not affected. On the other hand, if pressure in the sample chamber is in the molecular range, as is required by the second equation, the viscous balance provided by the sample chamber to pump viscous flow is lost. Under these circumstances an increase in viscosity decreases flow into the sample chamber. If flow decreases and pump speed does not change, then pressure will drop. A decrease in pressure in the sample chamber will reduce pressure in the ionization chamber and ultimately lower the measurement. In summary, with molecular flow there is no viscosity-dependent resistance between sample chamber and pump; consequently, viscous balancing is not possible. When flows are maintained in the viscous region, viscous balancing occurs, and the pressure profile across the sampling system is maintained and is independent of viscosity.

This presents a conundrum. Viscous flow in the sampling system maintains pressures in the sampling chamber that are not viscosity-dependent. However,

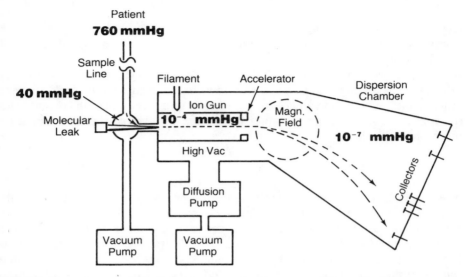

FIGURE 11.2   *Pressure gradients in a mass spectrometer. Two vacuum systems are required: a low vacuum to aspirate the sample to the spectrometer, and a high vacuum to sort and make possible the accurate detection of the ion fragments. The transitional flow between the two at the molecular leak must be designed carefully to ensure accurate results.*

sample flow into the ionization chamber requires pressure in the sample chamber to be in the molecular range. There are really two answers to that problem. First, there are porous materials that extend the range of molecular flow up to 40 to 50 mm Hg.[2] Thus, viscosity balancing is realized on the sample side and molecular flow is realized on the ionization chamber side. Second, mass spectrometers now being used for monitoring have fast, automatic summing networks. These networks assume that all the component gases in a gas sample equal 100%, which enables some variation in sample chamber pressures to be well tolerated.

DIFFUSION PUMPS

In a mass spectrometer there are two vacuum systems (Figure 11.2): one handles the sample tubing and the other the mass spectrometer. The vacuum requirements for the sampling tubing are much less demanding than those for the spectrometer proper and can be satisfied by a simple, rotary, oil-sealed mechanical pump, which works well in the micron pressure range. The mass spectrometer, on the other hand, requires much lower pressures, and the mechanical pump must be supported by a different pumping mechanism. Historically, diffusion pumps were first used and worked best in the molecular region (Figure 11.3).[4] Vapor from a boiler jets into the vacuum, trapping gas molecules and compressing them so that they can be removed by the mechanical pump. A series of nozzles may be required. Early pumps used mercury. Today many oils are available that have vapor pressures in the 10^{-6} to 10^{-8} mm Hg range at 25°C and work well. Baffles are used to prevent oil vapors from getting to the dispersion section of the mass spectrometer and thus minimize maintenance.

A second type of pump requires ionization of the resident gas molecules.[5] It has been known for some time that low-pressure gas-discharge tubes such as fluorescent and neon lights lose internal pressure with use to the point where pressure is too low to support the discharge and the tube fails. In vacuum technology this effect is used to advantage and involves several mechanisms. Gaseous ions simply adhere or are absorbed on internal surfaces. The usual implementation uses a cathode and anode; positive ions impact the cathode and cause material to be sputtered off that will trap or absorb gas molecules when condensation occurs. A judicious choice of material here may enhance the absorbing capability. Gas ions may combine chemically with any of the

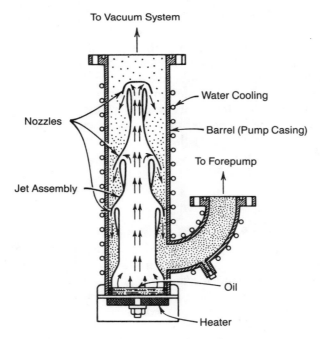

FIGURE 11.3   *Oil diffusion pump. Oil vapor jetting through the nozzles compresses resident gas molecules, making it possible to remove them with a mechanical or fore pump. Although these pumps are described as diffusion pumps, the mechanism actually involves molecular collisions and might more appropriately be called impact pumps. (Reproduced with permission from Guthrie A: Vacuum Technology. New York, John Wiley, 1963.)*

above materials. In general, any action that removes gas molecules will decrease pressure and increase pumping action. In the mass spectrometer ion pumps absorb gas molecules into noble metal plates. These saturate and must be changed at 6- to 12-month intervals.[6]

Instrument Specificity

Up to this point, we have assumed that the mass fragments generated in the ionization chamber are simply gas molecules with an electron stripped off, *e.g.,* CO_2^+ or N_2^+. In actuality, there are these species and other fragments as well. Any of the fragments are candidates for tracking because each bears a fixed relationship to the parent gas as long as the ionization conditions are unchanged. Among the gases of interest during anesthesia, carbon dioxide and nitrous oxide have approximately the same mass at 44. This problem might be resolved by electing to measure the NO^+ signal at mass 30. In practice, this is difficult because of variable overlap from the strong peaks of O_2^+ at 32 and N_2^+ at 28. A better solution has proven to be measuring the C^+ fragment at mass 12 for carbon dioxide and subtracting the result from the signal at mass 44. The remainder at mass 44, then, is the signal from N_2O^+.

Anesthetic agents have also proven to be a challenge. Most mass spectrometers cover a mass range from approximately 2 to 136; however, the mass of halothane is 197.4, enflurane 184.5, and isoflurane 184.5. Fortunately, measuring ion fragments provides a solution; under controlled conditions, each of these anesthetics produces fragments at mass 67 and mass 51. The ratio of 67/51 is different for each agent and thus can be used for identification (Table 11.1). After identifying the agent the electronic gain can be appropriately set at mass 67 for measurement.

SAMPLING

For shared systems, there are two ways of sampling. In one* gas samples are continuously aspirated through long tubes at a fixed flow of 4 ml/sec. A rotary sample selector sequentially samples gas from each of the sampling tubes. With this design the flow rate into the analyzer is the same as the sampling flow. Dwell time (the time for sampling per station) can be adjusted by either the number of breaths or the number of seconds.

In a second system** analysis flow (3 ml/sec) is twice the rate of sampling

---

*Perkin Elmer Corporation
 Applied Science Division
 2771 North Garey Avenue
 Pomona, CA 91767

**Allegheny International Medical Technology
 897 Fee Fee Road
 St. Louis, MO 63043

Table 11.1 The Mass Weight Ratio and Gain Requirements Used to Analyze Anesthetic Gases[3]

Gas	Mass Weight Ratio 67/51	Gain Requirements at 67
Halothane	7.5	1.00
Enflurane	1.45	2.67
Isoflurane	0.44	0.92

flow (1.4 ml/sec).[3] In this way the sample tubing can also serve as storage area. At the lower flow a 20-sec profile is continuously stored in the sample line. When the sample lines are switched to the analyzer, doubling the flow enables analysis in approximately 7 sec (Figure 11.4).

SHARED MASS SPECTROMETERS

Because some mass spectrometers are too expensive to be used as freestanding dedicated instruments, several systems have been introduced that serve multiple

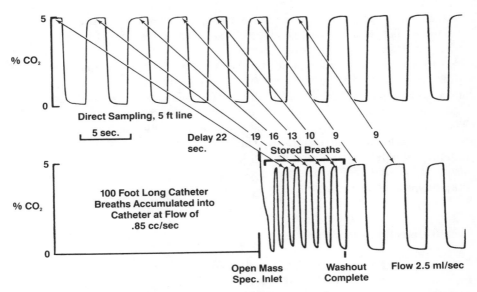

FIGURE 11.4 *Storage of gas samples in the sampling line. Dwell time can be reduced by storing patient gas in the sampling line at a reduced flow. Increasing flow during analysis makes it possible to analyze the stored breaths faster than they actually occurred, thus dwell time is reduced. (Reproduced with permission from Ozanne GM, Young WG, Mazzei WJ, et al: Multipatient anesthetic mass spectrometry: Rapid analysis of data stored in long catheters. Anesthesiology 55:62–70, 1980. Courtesy J.B. Lippincott and Company, Hagerstown, MD.)*

patients simultaneously. This requires a centrally located mass spectrometer with tubing from each patient to a valving mechanism and then to the mass spectrometer. The advantage of such a system is that it is economic. The disadvantage is that it is discontinuous; the instrument must cycle through all patients before returning to the first for analysis of another sample. Because the capillary tubes carrying the gas samples often have to bridge 100 feet or more, dwell times are long. When the instrument fails, all patients are affected. In order to sidestep this problem and increase safety, some manufacturers have incorporated sidestream infrared capnometers into the mass spectrometer system.

Dwell Time Algorithms

For shared systems, measurement criteria that control dwell time, or the time for sampling and analysis per station, must be developed. Two approaches have been described, both starting with the carbon dioxide waveform to determine inspiration and expiration. In one approach[7] increasing carbon dioxide followed by a plateau indicates expiration. A decreasing signal followed by zero or close to zero indicates inspiration. The time at which the maximum minimum carbon dioxide signals are measured is used to trigger the measurement for all gases. This information is confirmed in a second breath before a value is displayed and before the monitor switches to the next station (patient).

In another system[7] a more dynamic approach is used. Two thresholds are used to identify inspiratory and expiratory efforts. These thresholds are self-adjusting. As the waveform increases, so do the thresholds. The logic is that an increasing signal that crosses both thresholds is expiration and a decreasing signal that crosses both thresholds is inspiration. The maximum after surpassing 75% will be the expiratory value and the minimum after becoming lower than the 25% level will be the inspiratory value. This dynamic approach is considered reliable enough that only one breath need be analyzed. However, this system also makes it possible for the operator to control dwell time by selecting either time or number of breaths.

Breath Detection Algorithms

Inspiration and expiration are distinguished by carbon dioxide values. In one implementation both time and carbon dioxide are used.[3] For example, the algorithm requires that, in time, the peak value (*i.e.*, end-tidal carbon dioxide) follows a minimal value by more than 0.75 sec. Assuming an inspiratory-to-expiratory ratio of 1:1, this filters out respiratory frequencies greater than 40 breaths/min. In addition, the decrease in end-tidal carbon dioxide must be at least 7 mm Hg and be within 3 mm Hg of that for the preceding breath. A second breath is analyzed to confirm the first. The computer will choose the peak with the higher end-tidal carbon dioxide and display the concentrations of all gases at that time. If no carbon dioxide is detected within 5 sec, gas from the next station is analyzed. This eliminates samples from breath rates slower than 6/min when the I:E is 1:1. If carbon dioxide is sensed but the signal does not meet the criteria for breath detection, dwell time could be extended to 15 seconds.

Algorithms have their limitations. For example, the dual threshold algorithm does not prevent cardiogenic oscillations from being analyzed as capnograms.[8] The reported value for the expired carbon dioxide, respiratory rate, and inspiratory carbon dioxide may all be in error. Any event causing a dip in the plateau, *i.e.,* decreasing the signal to less than 25%, will satisfy the algorithm and may cause erroneous results. In addition to cardiogenic oscillations, such waveforms could come from artifact.

Confusion may be prevented by continually checking the scaled capnogram against the displayed values. Further, inspiratory-to-expiratory ratios are often computed from the capnogram, but these are only estimates because expiratory flow starts before the upstroke of the capnogram. In addition, as mentioned earlier, high airway pressure alters transit time and distorts inspiratory-to-expiratory ratios.

In addition to processing algorithms, the quality of information can be safeguarded in other ways. For example, if no information is sensed within a set time, an alarm will be activated because either apnea or a disconnection may have occurred. If values are beyond the physiologic range, the instrument should alert a user to the possibility of a calibration problem. Physiologic reactions require time; therefore, consecutive values should not change drastically. Large instantaneous changes usually indicate a technical problem.

SUMMING NETWORKS

The summing networks used by most mass spectrometers assume that all inspired and expired gases are being measured. Therefore, discounting water vapor, the fractional parts should equal 1 and the partial pressures should equal atmospheric pressure. When all gases are being measured, technical requirements are simplified, and adding the results provides a quick check for reliability. However, when this is not the case, problems can occur. For example, adding an aerosol propellant to the breathing gas produces some unexpected results.[9,10]

The first observation is that adding any foreign gas to the breathing gas dilutes the other constituent gases. Thus, the concentrations of all the gases decrease. If the foreign gas is not measured by the spectrometer, the concentrations that are reported will be erroneously high. If the foreign gas has mass fragments that are detected, they might be identified as an agent and concentration of that agent will be reported as falsely high. At the same time, this would lower the concentrations reported for the other gases (*e.g.,* oxygen or carbon dioxide), but transiently and unpredictably. Mass spectrometers have set limits for maximal concentrations; exceeding these limits also may produce erroneous results.[11] The best way to avoid these problems is to administer drugs or foreign gases at a time when the mass spectrometer is not sampling or to ignore the results at those times.

Helium presents a different type of problem, specifically for spectrometers with an ion pump. Ion pumps work by absorbing gases into noble metal plates, which may be a slow process for helium. Consequently, residual helium may affect the reading for the next station and cause erroneously low concentrations to be reported for the other gases.[6]

Water Vapor

Inspired gases are usually dry, but expired gases are saturated with water vapor at body temperature. Mass spectrometers have two problems with water vapor. First, condensation in the sample tubing may block sample flow. Second, water vapor is absorbed by the plastic tubes but will be washed out later when gases of lower humidity pass through. Water is absorbed even in metal tubes heated to eliminate condensation. Regardless of the type of sampling tube, the response to water vapor is delayed. This effect has been eliminated by filtering vapor from the gas sample before it enters the tubing and by analyzing as if the gas were dry.

The Use of Sums and Ratios

Although water vapor is eliminated from on-line measurement, its influence on gas composition must be considered; after all, expired gas is 6% water vapor. Mass spectrometers compensate for water vapor in the following way. A summing network assumes that all the fractional concentrations add up to 100% or the partial pressures add up to atmospheric pressure. The user can input information on gases that are known but not measured or that do not change during breathing. For example, during inspiration the partial pressure of water vapor can be set to 10 mm Hg during expiration to 47 mm Hg. In these cases the total pressure for all the other gases would be 750 mm Hg during inspiration and 713 mm Hg during expiration. If one wishes to focus on alveolar concentrations for both inspired and expired gases, then the appropriate sum is 713 mm Hg. Also, if air were the subject gas, a fixed and unchanging value for argon (0.95% or 7 mm Hg) could be introduced.

The addition of summing networks to mass spectrometers has been an important factor in their wide acceptance. It has provided constant system sensitivity over long-term use in spite of changes that might otherwise disturb readings such as flow restrictions, pressure, or viscosity.

Quadrupole Mass Filter

The magnetic sector and quadrupole instruments are similar in that both require a high vacuum because the MFP must be long compared with the chamber dimensions and because the separation scheme requires that the particles be charged. The principles used for separation, however, are quite different. The quadrupole is really a mass filter that depends on the influence of a combined DC and radio frequency field (Figure 11.5). Four parallel rods are designed so that the tuning of the combined fields will result in particles of only one type traversing the longitudinal axis and ending up at the detector. The trajectory of all others is such that they strike one of the four rods and are removed from the ion beam. Changing the voltages in a controlled way makes it possible to scan the mass spectrum. This can be done in a few milliseconds.

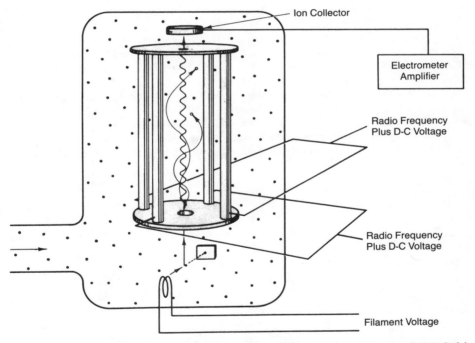

FIGURE 11.5 *Quadrupole mass filter. Tuning the radio frequency and DC fields causes particles of one mass to traverse the longitudinal axis and strike the collector. All others strike one of the four rods and are eliminated from the ion beam. Scanning and sampling the voltage in a controlled way makes detection of all charged particles possible. Repetitive scanning and sampling provides continuous monitoring. (Reproduced with permission from Steinherz HA, Redhead PA: Ultrahigh vacuum. Sci Am 206:78–90, 1962. Copyright © 1962 by Scientific American, Inc. All rights reserved.)*

Sampling the collector output at appropriate times in the scan makes it possible to measure the component masses. Scanning and sampling repetitively provide continuous monitoring.

REFERENCES

1. Hill NC: Introduction to Mass Spectrometry. London, Heyden, 1966
2. Fowler KT: The respiratory mass spectrometer. Phys Med Biol 14:185–199, 1969
3. Ozanne GM, Young WG, Mazzei WJ, et al: Multipatient anesthetic mass spectrometry: Rapid analysis of data stored in long catheters. Anesthesiology 55:62–70, 1981
4. Guthrie A: Vacuum Technology. New York, Wiley, 1963
5. Barrington AE: High Vacuum Engineering. Englewood Cliffs, NJ, Prentice Hall, 1963
6. Severinghaus JW: Monitoring anesthetic and respiratory gases, in Blitt CD (ed): Monitoring in Anesthesia and Critical Care Medicine. New York, Churchill Livingstone, 1985
7. Gravenstein JS, Gravenstein N, van der Aa JJ, et al: Pitfalls with mass spectrometry in clinical anesthesia. Int J Comput Monit 1:27–34, 1984
8. May WS, Heavner JE, McWhoter D, et al: Capnography in the Operating Room. New York, Raven, 1985
9. Gillbe CE, Heneghan CPH, Branthwaite MA: Respiratory mass spectrometry during general anaesthesia. Br J Anaesth 53:103–108, 1981
10. Gravenstein N, Theisen GJ, Knudsen AK: Misleading mass spectrometer reading caused by an aerosol propellant. Anesthesiology 62:70–72, 1985
11. McCleary U Jr: Potential effects of an unknown gas on mass spectrometer readings. Anesthesiology 63:724–725, 1985

Chapter 12

Gas Sampling

SIDESTREAM SAMPLING

Mass spectrometers, Raman devices, and many infrared instruments use sidestream sampling (Figure 12.1). Gas is sampled at flow rates between 50 and 240 ml/min. A typical infrared instrument has two flow rate settings: 50 ml/min or 150 ml/min. The sample is aspirated from a lightweight T-piece on the airway through 5 to 10 feet of tubing to a remote optical bench where the gas is analyzed. The size and weight of this T-piece connection is a major advantage of sidestream monitors. Some breathing circuit suppliers have incorporated the sample tube into the design of the breathing circuit.

Condensed water and secretions from the patient can accumulate in the sample tubing and potentially interfere with flow and also disrupt measurement in other ways. Most instruments have a way of preventing water from entering the sample cell, such as an absorbent, a water trap, or tubing with a very high permeability for water vapor. Tubing with some unusual characteristics is made from Nafion (Dupont), a perfluorinated ion exchange polymer. This material, prepared with cation exchange sites, which make it permeable to many cations and to polar solvents such as water, quickly transports water from the inside of the tube where water vapor pressure is high to the outside where water vapor pressure is relatively low.

Another technique is a reverse flush, which is triggered either manually or by an excessive pressure drop across the sample tube. Infection control, however, argues against this practice because of the danger of bacterial spores being forced back into the patient circuit from the permanent parts of the measuring system. To back up the water trap, at least one instrument has a high-suction purge that clears most sample tube blockages.[1]

How to dispose of sample gas after it has been measured has been the topic of much discussion. Simply discharging the sample into the room is not satisfactory because the sample contains nitrous oxide, anesthetic, and possibly airborne bacteria from the patient or from the instrument. Returning the sample to the breathing circuit does not solve the problem because of the possibility, again, of adding infectious agents from the permanent parts of the measuring system. The recommended solution is to discharge the sample into the hospital scavenging system. Most instruments have a port for connecting the scavenging

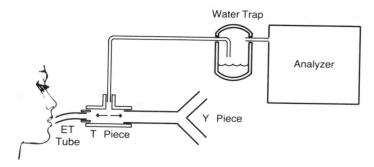

FIGURE 12.1   *Sidestream sampling. Patient gases are aspirated at a controlled flow from the breathing circuit, near the endotracheal tube (ET). The trap prevents water from getting into the analyzer and interfering with the analysis.*

tubing. The scavenging tubing may add significant resistance to the system and change the pressure in the sample chamber. This could change the calibration. Thus, calibration should always be done with the scavenging tubing in place, or sample chamber pressure should be measured for appropriate corrections. Some instruments automatically compensate for pressure changes in the sample chamber.

One way to minimize the possibility of cross-contamination is to use a bacterial filter between patient and instrument, which is an option on some instruments. Such an addition, however, may add resistance, may change the pressure in the sample chamber, and may alter response time. These things must be considered when a filter is used. One other consideration with water traps is the need for appropriate infection control measures when water traps are emptied because of potentially infectious material.

Sample Flow Rate

Because sample gas is removed from the airway, the relationship between the amount of gas removed and the patient's requirements must be considered, particularly in a closed-circuit system. If fresh gas flow rate ever becomes less than sample flow rate, air might leak into the system, the gas delivered to the patient may change, and the capnogram and end-tidal values may be affected.[2] Clearly, fresh gas flow must satisfy the patient's requirements and the sampling requirements.[3] For this, the system must be tight.

The ventilation of neonates requires a small tidal volume and a high respiratory rate. The small tidal volume argues for lower sampling flow rates. This makes measuring higher respiratory rates more difficult because of the relationship between flow and response time. For low rates of flow, more time is needed to wash out the sample cuvette, which prolongs the time constant. Again, measuring systems with appropriate time constants even at low rates of flow should be a requirement. In contrast, if the sample flow rate in a partial rebreathing system is too high, fresh gas may become mixed with the gas sample during the expiratory phase [4-6]; this may distort the plateau and possibly mask the true end-tidal value.

Sampling Site

In addition to sample flow rate, the position of the sampling catheter relative to the source of fresh gas in a Bain or Mapleson D circuit is important. Sampling from a site close to the endotracheal tube and away from the source of fresh gas keeps fresh gas from being entrained with sample gas.[6] This is supported by a bench study designed to investigate the influence of fresh gas flow, sample flow, and expiratory flow on measured carbon dioxide.[4] A computer model for this circuit was devised and later verified.[7,8]

In a similar way, air can be entrained with sample gas. For example, if the fitting between the sample tubing and the capnograph leaks, entrainment of air during exhalation causes the early part of the capnogram to be erroneously low.[9] Remember, there is a pressure drop across the sample tubing and, during part of the respiratory cycle, the pressure at the point of connection to the instrument is less than atmospheric. During inhalation, airway pressure increases on the mechanically ventilated patient. This increase is instantly transmitted along the sampling catheter and, because pressure is now greater than atmospheric, the leak stops and the capnogram rises.

The time relationship between these events is determined by flow rate, length of tubing and respiratory rate. It is also important to remember that ambient air can be entrained when a noncuffed endotracheal tube is used with a hanging bellows ventilator (which creates a negative pressure). This diluent effect occurs at the distal end of the endotracheal tube and, therefore, will influence mainstream as well as sidestream analyzers. The important point is that capnograms can be distorted either by improper positioning of the sample catheter, by leaks, or by inappropriate fresh gas flows in both closed and partial rebreathing systems.

Water Trap

Instrument design can influence capnographic results in yet another interesting and unpredictable way. Recently an artifact in the upstroke of the capnogram was reported to result from the combination of high airway pressure (greater than 30 cm H_2O) and a water trap with a large volume.[10] A two-compartment model for this problem was constructed (Figure 12.2). One compartment consists of gases accumulated over time that contain carbon dioxide; the other compartment is sample gas from the patient that is being exchanged continuously. With high airway pressure, gas in the water trap is significantly com-

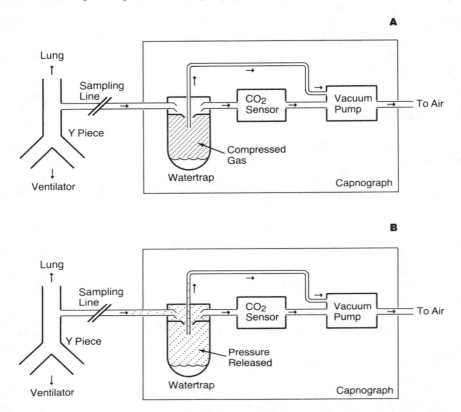

FIGURE 12.2 *Capnogram artifact and water traps. Large water traps (>10 ml) produce artifact which has its origins in the phases of respiration and whose appearance depends on respiratory rate. (A) At the end of inspiration, the system is pressurized at peak airway pressure (P_{aw}) and filled with fresh gas, except for the lower part of the water trap, which holds a gas mixture containing carbon dioxide (shaded). (B) At the beginning of expiration, P_{aw} decreases to baseline. The pressurized gas mixture in the lower part of the water trap expands and some flows into the sampling tube, the carbon dioxide content of which is eventually detected by the capnograph. Its appearance on the capnogram depends on the respiratory rate. (Reprinted with permission from the International Anesthesia Research Society from van Genderingen HR, Gravenstein N: Capnogram artifact during high airway pressures caused by a water trap. Anesth Analg 66:185–187, 1987.)*

pressed. For a patient on a ventilator, airway pressure falls quickly during exhalation. The decrease has an immediate effect on the water trap—the carbon dioxide-containing gas expands and enters the first compartment. If the delay is such that inspiratory gas from a previous breath was about to be analyzed, the gas sample will be contaminated with a small amount of carbon dioxide. The problem does not occur as long as the volume of the water trap is less than 10 ml.

Effect on Inspiratory and Expiratory Phases of the Capnogram

One other interesting influence of varying airway pressure is that it affects flow in the sample tubing. Increasing pressure will increase flow. Changes in airway pressure are instantly transmitted across the sampling catheter and can influence the time relationship between the inspiratory and expiratory phases of the capnogram. This is not the same as the inspiratory-to-expiratory ratio, which depends on flow reversal in the airways, not the concentration of carbon dioxide.[11]

MAINSTREAM SAMPLING

Early attempts at monitoring recognized the advantages of measuring carbon dioxide directly as the patient exhaled (Figure 12.3). However, these devices were too large and cumbersome to be practical. Modern technology, however, has solved this problem and provided monitors that more easily fit into the clinical environment.[12] To connect the mainstream system to a patient, an adapter can be placed at the endotracheal tube (Figure 12.4). Two sizes of adapters usually are available, one for adult and pediatric applications and one for neonates. These breathe-through adapters define the volume of gas being

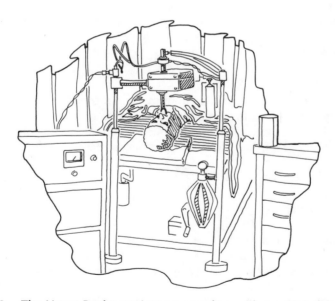

FIGURE 12.3 *The Liston-Becker mainstream analyzer. The mainstream or breathe-through analyzer was similar in design to the NDIR double-beam, positive-filter capnometer shown in Figure 10.5 (Adapted with permission from Elam JA, Brown EI, Ten Pas RH: Carbon dioxide homeostasis during anesthesia. Instrumentation. Anesthesiology 16: 876, 1955.)*

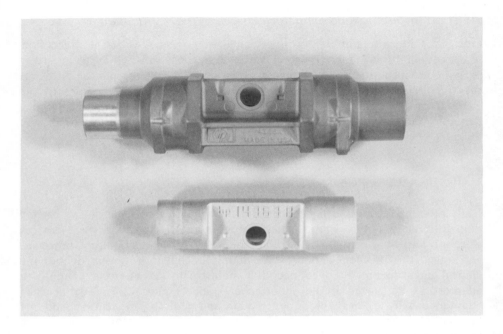

FIGURE 12.4   *Airway adapters for a mainstream capnometer. The adult/pediatric adapter has a dead space of 15 cc, and the neonate adapter, 2 cc. Mainstream adapters should have low resistance to flow and should not increase the work of breathing. (Courtesy of Hewlett Packard.)*

monitored and make it possible to monitor the concentration of carbon dioxide continuously throughout the breathing cycle. A requirement for these airway adapters is that they must be sterilizable for infection control. One recently introduced capnograph has included both mainstream and sidestream capability.[13]

Conditions of Analysis

Using the sidestream approach, measurements are made at a flow rate that is constant, in a chamber that is at room temperature, and on a gas that is saturated with water vapor. Although circumstances can alter these conditions—mucus, scavenging system connections, or change in room temperature—the measurement is reasonably well controlled.

With mainstream sampling, the patient and the mode of ventilation—not the capnometer—control the analytical circumstances. For example, expired gas is usually 33°C and saturated with water vapor, and, at the end of expiration, pressure is atmospheric. In addition, the measurements of end-tidal carbon dioxide and inspiratory minimum carbon dioxide are made at the ends of their respective phases when flow is at or near zero.

Pressures

Pressures change in the patient's circuit in a way that is related to the patient's ventilation. Inspiratory pressures can be as high as 40 to 50 cm H_2O. This can influence the inspiratory minimum carbon dioxide through compression and line broadening, but this is usually a small effect. At the end of exhalation, the pressure generally is close to atmospheric. Exceptions, of course, are when positive end-expiratory (PEEP) and continuous positive airway (CPAP) pressures are applied.

PEEP and CPAP compress the end expired gas, which increases the end-tidal carbon dioxide. In addition, pressure increases the line broadening effect, which also increases the measurement. In these and similar circumstances, the displayed value will overestimate the end-tidal carbon dioxide, but rarely by more than 3 mm Hg. When correcting for these effects is important, use the following equation:

$$P_{ACT} = P_{DSP} \times \frac{(CF)_2}{(CF)_1} \times \frac{P_a}{P_a + PEEP}$$

where P_{ACT} = the corrected value for the end-tidal carbon dioxide,

$\quad$ P_{DSP} = the displayed value,

$\quad$ $(CF)_2$ = the line broadening correction factor in the presence of PEEP,

$\quad$ $(CF)_1$ = the correction in its absence

$\quad$ P_a = atmospheric pressure

PEEP = the positive end-expiratory pressure.

For example, when the displayed value is 50 mm Hg and PEEP is 15 cm H_2O, altitude corrections interpolated from Figure 12.5 provide the following:

$$P_{ACT} = 50 \times \frac{1.018}{1.025} \times \frac{720.0}{720.0 + 11.11}$$
$$= 48.90 \text{ mm Hg.}$$

The above treatment assumes a line broadening or altitude correction in processing the measured values. Setting that correction makes it possible to correct for the significant influence of altitude. For example, measurements in Denver, CO (atmospheric pressure = 630 mm Hg) would read 7.5% less than in Boston, MA where the atmospheric pressure = 760 mm Hg (Figure 12.5). The influence of weather fronts or daily changes in barometric pressure is generally considered to be small. One study indicates that in Bristol, England, on only two days out of the studied year did pressure change by more than

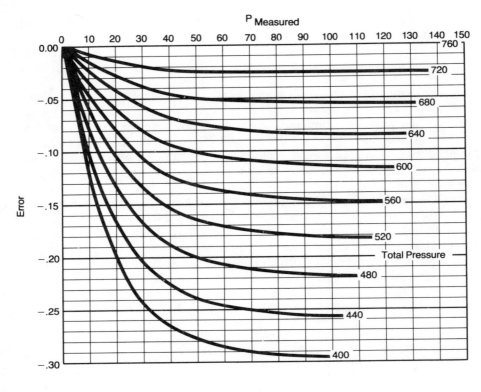

$$E = \frac{P \text{ measured} - P \text{ actual}}{P \text{ actual}}$$

FIGURE 12.5 *Pressure broadening effect. Calibration curves are usually determined at a total pressure of 760 mm Hg. Decreasing total pressure causes a decrease in carbon dioxide signal. the measured carbon dioxide ($P_{measured}$) will be less than the true carbon dioxide (P_{actual}). Error as defined in the figure will be negative for decreasing total pressure. For example, if $P_{measured}$ = 50 mm Hg and the total pressure is 600 mm Hg, the E = −0.10, $P_{actual} = \frac{P_{measured}}{1 + E} = \frac{50}{0.9} \cdot P_{actual} = 55.5$.*

2.93 mm Hg.[14] Of course, this depends on local conditions and could vary significantly from one location to another. Even so, a change of 10 mm Hg can have a line broadening influence of only 0.5 to 1.0% in the physiological range, depending on altitude.

As indicated earlier, the pressure broadening effect is dependent on instrument design (see Chapter 10). Other published results indicate a 0.8% change for a 1% change in pressure in another mainstream instrument.[15]

Response Time

Because carbon dioxide is detected as it emerges from the patient, the measurement is nearly instantaneous and high-fidelity waveforms are obtained. The time constant, however, may not differ significantly from that with sidestream analyzers.[1,11] Sidestream instruments with high rates of sampling flow and cuvettes with small volumes may have very fast response times.

Infection Control

The transducer is isolated from patient gases and so is not a major factor in infection control. The airway adapter, however, must be sterilizable.

Flow Control

Flow is controlled by the patient and the ventilator, not by the analyzer. This eliminates the need for a flow control system involving pumps, flow meters, control valves, and pressure transducers.

Water Vapor

Expired gases are assumed to have a temperature of 33°C and to be saturated with water vapor. The water vapor has a slight line broadening effect, which is usually automatically taken into consideration in the processing.[12] Warming of the adapter by the transducer prevents condensation, which minimizes maintenance.

Processing Algorithms

Although the expiratory carbon dioxide waveform is usually described in classically ideal terms, the circumstances in monitoring carbon dioxide in the airway are not always ideal. Artifact can be generated by valves opening and closing, by the accidental compression of the breathing circuit, or by a surgeon leaning on the patient's chest. In addition, patient-related circumstances may cause unusual waveforms, *e.g.*, fighting the ventilator or cardiogenic oscillations. One of the challenges is to process this information accurately so that only the desired information is extracted. This processing is one of the significant contributions of programmable microprocessors.

The objective is to select values of end-tidal and minimal inspiratory carbon dioxide and a respiratory rate that are not influenced by artifact. The first step is to see if the waveform reflects respiration. This can be done by dividing the waveform into three zones (low, medium, and high) by using appropriate filtering and bracketing procedures. The signal must progress from low to medium to high and then from high to medium to low; in other words, the signal must go up and down in an orderly fashion. In addition, the signal must remain in each zone for a particular amount of time; this prevents fast transient values from being analyzed. This time of residency depends on respiratory rate, the time being briefer at higher rates. Once these conditions are satisfied, the waveform is accepted as a respiratory waveform and analysis begins. The maximal value in the high zone is considered end-tidal carbon dioxide and the lowest value in the low zone is the minimal inspiratory value. Respiratory rate is calculated as the average of the preceding six-breath intervals. This describes the algorithm used by one manufacturer (Hewlett Packard); others use different algorithms that are also satisfactory.

Operational Considerations

As with all techniques, mainstream sampling has its limitations. It is usually used on intubated patients or can be applied using a face mask. Great progress has been made in reducing the size of the transducer, but it is still larger and weighs more than the sidestream sampling tube and T-piece. In the operating room the mainstream assembly can be supported by a bracket along with the rest of the breathing circuit; in the intensive care unit the articulating support arm on the ventilator is helpful. A flexible tube placed between the endotracheal tube and the airway adapter reduces the direct influence of the transducer mass but can only be used when additional dead space can be tolerated.

Accumulated water is not a problem because the transducer warms the airway, which prevents condensation. However, when mucus and secretions accumulate, the artificial airway must be changed; a status display usually indicates when such conditions require attention. Placing an elbow between the endotracheal tube and the airway deflects the secretions from the adapter and extends the time between changes.

Airway Adapters

In the past, some airway adapters required the use of disposable plastic couplers; if these couplers are reused, wear might cause a disconnection.[16] Therefore, disposable couplers should not be reused, and their cost, as well as that of all supplies, should be factored into the cost of operation.[17] A disconnection should activate monitor alarms or should be detected visually on the display when the waveform disappears. Most airways are now designed as one piece.

Transducer-Airway Fit

Infrared transducers, which are designed to snap onto the airway adapter, may loosen with time because of wear. A partial separation can cause an abrupt change in end-tidal carbon dioxide, which may be misinterpreted as a decrease of cardiac output or air embolism.[18] To prevent this possibility, the transducer should be strapped to the adapter. Interpreting a sudden change in a value should be guided by the fact that technical problems generally produce abrupt changes, whereas physiology changes slowly. For instance, air embolism usually produces an exponential decay, which would be seen in a trend display or recording.

Rugged Design

Mainstream transducers are complex: a number of optical and electrical components are packaged inside a relatively small, but usually shock-resistant housing. Usually mounted on an airway adapter, the transducer may be in some danger of falling or being dropped onto the floor at the end of monitoring or during an emergency. Susceptibility to damage should be investigated thoroughly.

In summary, capnography has produced two sampling techniques that have received wide acceptance. Sidestream analyzers use a lightweight adapter that makes possible the aspiration of airway gas through small lumen tubing to a remote analyzer. Suitable flow rates and a tight system must be maintained to provide acceptable response times and waveform fidelity. Some delay may be experienced because of sample transport time. Calibration typically requires the periodic use of flowing gases. Mainstream analyzers use a heavier patient interface but have no time delay. They use wide-lumen tubing and generally can be calibrated using built-in sealed gas cells.

REFERENCES

1. Anonymous: Evaluation: Carbon dioxide monitors. ECRI Health Dev 15:255–271, 1986
2. Epstein RA, Reznik AM, Epstein MAF: Determinants of distortions in CO_2 catheter sampling systems: A mathematical model. Respir Physiol 41:127–136, 1980
3. Huffman LM, Riddle RT: Mass spectrometer and/or capnograph use during low-flow, closed circuit anesthesia administration (letter to the editor). Anesthesiology 66:439–440, 1987
4. Gravenstein N, Lampotang S, Beneken JEW: Factors influencing capnography in the Bain circuit. J Clin Monit 1:6–10, 1985
5. Kaplan RF, Paulus DA: Error in sampling of exhaled gases. Anesth Analg 62:955–956, 1983
6. Brandom BW, Cook DR: Error in sampling of exhaled gases. Anesth Analg 62:956, 1983
7. Beneken JEW, Gravenstein N, Gravenstein JS, et al: Capnography and the Bain circuit I: A computer model. J Clin Monit 1:103–113, 1985

8. Beneken JEW, Gravenstein N, Lampotang S, et al: Capnography and the Bain circuit II: Validation of a computer model. J Clin Monit 3:165–177, 1987
9. Martin M, Zupan J, Benumof JL: Unusual end-tidal CO_2 waveform. Anesthesiology 66:712–713, 1987
10. van Genderingen HR, Gravenstein N: Capnogram artifact during high airway pressures caused by a water trap. Anesth Analg 66:185–187, 1987
11. Brunner JX, Westenskow DR: How carbon dioxide analyzer rise time affects the accuracy of carbon dioxide measurements. J Clin Monit 4: 134, 1988
12. Solomon RJ: A reliable, accurate CO_2 analyzer for medical use. Hewlett Packard J 32:3–21, 1981
13. Tremper KK: Consumer report panel: Which capnometer should I buy. New York, Postgraduate Assembly in Anesthesiology Program, NYSSA, 1987, pp 110–111
14. Cormack RS, Powell JN: Improving the performance of the infrared carbon dioxide meter. Br J Anaesth 44:131–141, 1972
15. Olsson SG, Fletcher R, Jonson B, et al: Clinical studies of gas exchange during ventilatory support—a method using the Siemens–Elema CO_2 analyzer. Br J Anaesth 52:491–499, 1980
16. Lenoir RJ: Hewlett Packard HP47210A capnometer. Br J Anaesth 58:1204, 1986
17. Lenoir RJ: Hewlett Packard Model 47210A. Health Dev-ECRI 16: 219–220, 1987
18. Ornstein E: False positive abrupt decrease in $ETCO_2$ during craniotomy in the sitting position. Anesthesiology 62:542, 1985

Index

Page numbers in *italics* indicate figures; page numbers followed by t indicate tabular material.